ETHICS, CULTURE, AND PSYCHIATRY

International Perspectives

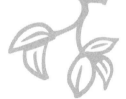

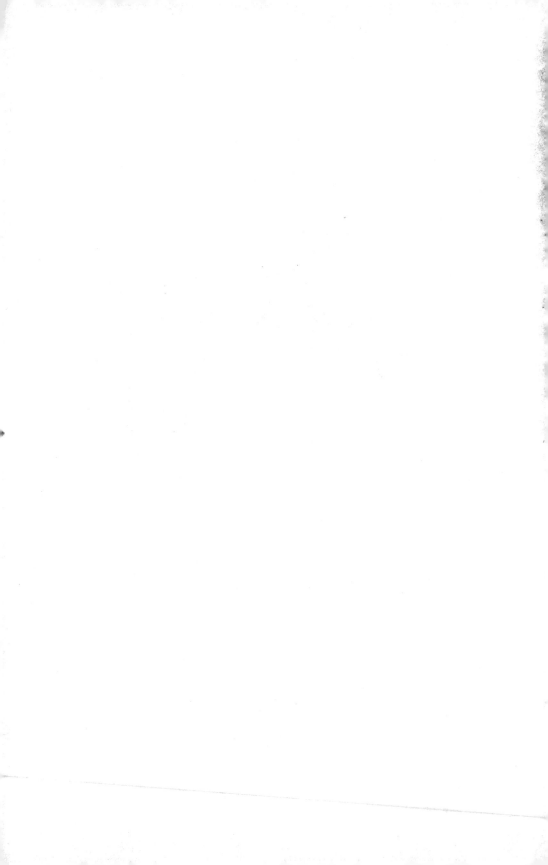

ETHICS, CULTURE, AND PSYCHIATRY

International Perspectives

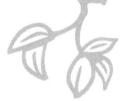

Edited by

Prof. Ahmed Okasha
Prof. Julio Arboleda-Flórez
Prof. Norman Sartorius

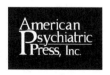

Washington, DC
London, England

Copyright © 2000 American Psychiatric Press, Inc.
ALL RIGHTS RESERVED
Manufactured in the United States of America on acid-free paper
03   02   01   00   4   3   2   1
First Edition

American Psychiatric Press, Inc.
1400 K Street, N.W., Washington, DC   20005
www.appi.org

Library of Congress Cataloging-in-Publication Data
Ethics, culture, and psychiatry / edited by Ahmed Okasha, Julio Arboleda-Florez, Norman Sartorius. — 1st ed.
      p. cm.
   Includes bibliographical references and index.
   ISBN 0-88048-999-5 (alk. paper)
   1. Psychiatric ethics.   2. Cultural psychiatry.   3. Psychiatry, Transcultural.   I. Ukashah, Ahmad.   II. Arboleda-Florez, J. (Julio), 1939- .   III. Sartorius, N.
      [DNLM: 1. Ethics, Medical.   2. Psychiatry.   3. Cross-Cultural Comparison.   WM 62 E833   2000]
   RC455.2E8   E836   2000
   616.89—dc21
                                                      99-040828

British Library Cataloguing in Publication Data
A CIP record is available from the British Library.

Contents

SECTION I

Ethics and Psychiatry Around the World

1

Prof. Norman Sartorius

2

Prof. Ahmed Okasha

3

Prof. Julio Arboleda-Flórez
Prof. David N. Weisstub

4

Prof. Juan J. López-Ibor, Jr.
Dr. M. Dolores Crespo

SECTION II

Overarching Issues

🌱 11

🌱 12

🌱 13

Contributors

Dr. Renato D. Alarcon
Professor and Vice Chairman, Department of Psychiatry and Behavioral Sciences, Emory University School of Medicine; and Chief, Mental Health Service Line, Veterans Administration Medical Center, Atlanta, Georgia

Prof. Julio Arboleda-Flórez
Member of the Ethics Committee of the World Psychiatric Association; and Professor and Head, Department of Psychiatry, Queen's University, Kingston, Ontario, Canada

Dr. M. Dolores Crespo
Associate Professor, Department of Psychiatry, Ramón y Cajal Hospital, University of Alcalá, Madrid, Spain

Prof. Dr. Hanfried Helmchen
Member of the Ethics Committee of the World Psychiatric Association; and Professor of Psychiatry, Department of Psychiatry, Free University of Berlin, Berlin, Germany

Dr. Marianne Kastrup
Medical Director, Rehabilitation and Research Centre for Torture Victims, Copenhagen, Denmark

Prof. Xiehe Liu
Professor and Director, Institute of Mental Health, West China University of Medical Sciences, Chengdu, China

Prof. Juan J. López-Ibor, Jr.
President of the World Psychiatric Association; and Head and Chairman, Department of Psychiatry, San Carlos Hospital, Complutense University, Madrid, Spain

Prof. R. Srinivasa Murthy
Professor of Psychiatry and Dean, National Institute of Mental Health and Neurosciences, Bangalore, India

Prof. Yoshibumi Nakane
Professor, Department of Neuropsychiatry, Nagasaki University School of Medicine, Nagasaki, Japan

Prof. Ahmed Okasha
Chairman of the Ethics Committee of the World Psychiatric Association (WPA) and President-Elect of the WPA; and Professor of Psychiatry and Director of the World Health Organization Collaborating Center for Training and Research in Mental Health, Institute of Psychiatry, Ain Shams University, Cairo, Egypt

Prof. Michael O. Olatawura
Professor of Psychiatry, University College Hospital, University of Ibadan, Ibadan, Nigeria

Prof. Mark Radford
Visiting Professor, Department of Neuropsychiatry, Nagasaki University School of Medicine, Nagasaki, Japan

Prof. Norman Sartorius
Past President of the World Psychiatric Association; and Professor of Psychiatry, Hospitaux Universitaires de Genève, Geneva, Switzerland

Prof. Dr. Dr. Jochen Vollmann
History of Medicine Institute, Free University of Berlin, Berlin, Germany

Prof. David N. Weisstub
Philippe Pinel Professor of Legal Psychiatry and Biomedical Ethics, Faculty of Medicine, University of Montreal, Montreal, Quebec, Canada

Preface

The idea of this book was born during a meeting with the leaders of the American Psychiatric Association, the American Psychiatric Press, Inc., and the Ethics Committee of the World Psychiatric Association (WPA). The group discussed how best to promote the use of the Declaration of Madrid (see the Appendix to this book), a consensus document adopted in 1996 by the General Assembly of the WPA.

The Declaration of Madrid was developed by the Ethics Committee of the WPA through a long process of consultation involving WPA member societies and individual experts, ethicists, psychiatrists, philosophers, and lawyers. The document contains a set of principles in the form of guidelines concerning ethical behavior in the practice of psychiatry.

It soon became obvious that the way in which the use of the declaration—and the application of the guidelines it contains—will be promoted will depend on the strength of the conviction of the Ethics Committee and of the General Assembly of the WPA that it is possible to formulate a set of principles that will be valid for all psychiatrists, regardless of the cultures to which they belong or in which they live and practice. Alternatively, perhaps there are as many sets of ethical principles as there are cultures, an approach that would mean a different way of proceeding in the years ahead.

Helman (1994) viewed culture as a set of guidelines, both explicit and implicit, that individuals inherit as members of a particular society and that indicate to them how to view the world, how to experience it emotionally, and how to behave in it in relation to other people, to supernatural forces or gods, and to the natural environment. These guidelines are transmitted to the next generation through the symbols, language, art, and ritual of culture. Ethics—through which what is good and what is bad are explored and which provide indications regarding behavior that enhances the good and minimizes the evil—could be expected to be culture specific, unless we were to postulate that in addition to belonging to individual cultures, humans also share a common culture.

To facilitate the exploration of this territory, we invited experts belonging to different cultures and familiar with the practice of psychiatry to write essays on ethical issues and psychiatry in the settings they knew well. We decided not to provide guidelines for the essays, because we thought the contributions would be richer and more emphatic about topics preoccupying psychiatrists in different lands if the writers were not constrained by guidelines.

Religious beliefs have a strong influence on ethics, morals, and deontological mistakes. Readers of this book shall discover, however, that although there are diverse cultures, only one human conscience, one human sense of responsibility, and one human moral obligation exist. There may be some agreement across all cultures on what is good, what is bad, and what should be denounced or praised.

We were impressed by the similarities among Indian, Chinese, Japanese, Latin American, and Arab cultures and by the denial of self for the sake of others and the devotion of the individual to the promotion of the group in these cultures. Individual autonomy is valued in Scandinavian, European, and American cultures but is not empowering for the traditional, family-centered societies in Arab, sub-Saharan African, Indian, and Japanese cultures. This difference may affect the use of involuntary admission, informed consent, and religious psychotherapy, among other practices, in traditional versus Western societies. In some cultures, traditional and religious healing have been combined with the most up-to-date psychopharmacological interventions.

We decided not to include a final chapter with conclusions about the ethical issues arising in the practice of psychiatry in the groups of countries covered in this book. One reason is that it is uncertain how closely the cultures are related in the groups of countries dealt with by the contributors and how representative the authors' views are of all psychiatrists working in the groups of countries described. Perhaps a more important reason for omitting a concluding chapter is that by bringing these materials together, we hope to stimulate and support, rather than close, the debate on ethical aspects of professional behavior in our own setting and in others—a debate animated by the wish to learn about the position of others and marked by respect for others' views and by a continuous search for a consensus on how to live together and make contributions to the well-being of people with mental illness, their families, and the family of humans on our planet.

Prof. Ahmed Okasha
Chairman of the Ethics Committee of the World Psychiatric Association (WPA)
President-Elect of the WPA
Professor of Psychiatry

*Director of the World Health Organization Collaborating Center for
Training and Research in Mental Health
Institute of Psychiatry, Ain Shams University
Cairo, Egypt*

Prof. Julio Arboleda-Flórez
*Member of the Ethics Committee of the WPA
Professor and Head, Department of Psychiatry
Queen's University
Kingston, Ontario, Canada*

Prof. Norman Sartorius
*Past President of the WPA
Professor of Psychiatry
Hospitaux Universitaires de Genève
Geneva, Switzerland*

Reference

Helman C: Culture, Health, and Illness: An Introduction for Health Professionals, 3rd Edition. Oxford, England, Butterworth-Heinemann, 1994, pp 6–9

SECTION I

Ethics and Psychiatry
Around the World

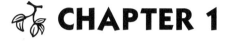 # CHAPTER 1

Ethics and the Societies of the World

Prof. Norman Sartorius

Two questions have led to the writing of this book. Both are easy to pose and difficult to answer. Both are important, because the responses to them will determine the organization of mental health care in many countries as well as international collaboration in the field of psychiatry.

The first of these questions is the following: Is there one set of rules that should govern the practice of psychiatry as a discipline, or are there as many sets of rules as there are societies? The second question is, If there is such a set of rules, what should we do to ensure that psychiatry as a discipline makes a significant contribution to societal good without helping the evil?

In seeking an answer to these two questions, I shall use the word *ethics* to describe the study of good and bad and of the general nature of morals in different societies; *deontology* to describe the study of standards governing the conduct of members of professions; *morals* to describe the standards of rectitude prevailing in a particular society at a given point in time; *ethical* to describe the accordance of an action with general or ideal standards of right and wrong, related to its contribution to the balance of good and bad in society; and *moral* to describe the accordance with standards prevailing in a given society at a given point in time.

The Context of Ethical Practice of Psychiatry

The answer to the first of the questions just stated will depend on, first, whether ethicists will be able to define the good and the bad in ways that can somehow be proven and, second, the likelihood that what is good and what is bad remain equal across time.

Over the years, various external criteria of validation of the definition of good and bad have been proposed. They include the following:

♦ The intervention of a divine being who has from time immemorial defined the good and the bad and ordered humankind to maintain the original distinction or be punished

♦ A reference to the evolutionary advantage that the acceptance of certain rules has for the species (the same justification has also been formulated somewhat differently regarding the survival and advancement of society as a whole)

♦ Historical analyses showing the immutability and repeated appearance of the same rules in different cultures and in different religious systems

♦ The consensus of the just and the wise, so wise that they could, despite their own anchors in time, see or sense the eternal truth

Through the ages, attempts have also been made to convince everyone that people of a particular country had discovered the way of distinguishing good and bad and that the moral behavior of professionals or citizens of belonging to that (usually economically or militarily strong) culture or country was in fact ethical behavior and that it was therefore justifiable and in the best interest of all to impose rules of moral behavior of professionals in that country on people in general or on professionals in all other countries in the world. Often the argument sounds plausible, drawing strength from the fact that the country putting forward a particular set of rules at a point of its maximum strength has, after all, achieved a position on the summit that might have been the consequence of observing the very rules proposed.

The immutability of the ideal definition of good and bad over time is also dependent on the orientation of the persons who argue about it. Those who hold the platonic view that somewhere there is a set of ideal models will be more easily convinced of the immunity of the definitions against the influences of time; those who hold the Aristotelian view and are not convinced that ideal models exist and who therefore search for the truth by examining all matters within their reach will probably argue that it is likely that the definition of good and bad changes over time, because, for example, of the changes in the capacity of humans to study historical development using modern methods of information exchange. The truth is probably in the middle: rules will change with time, but their changes are infrequent and reflect changes in ethical paradigms of society—in the same way that rules in science change with changes in the paradigms of science (Kuhn 1970).

Even if it were possible to produce an eternal and cross-culturally valid definition of good and bad, it would still be necessary to develop criteria for guidance in deciding which paths for achieving good and avoiding bad are acceptable. In Indian ethics, for example, happiness, health, survival, progeny, pleasure, calmness, friendship, knowledge, and truth are placed on the side of good—the highest good is the total harmony of the cosmic order—and misery and other opposites of the good things are considered bad (Bilimoria 1997). All people are expected to behave in a way that promotes the good and that does not lead to the production of bad things, because otherwise the order of the universe might be disturbed. However, there is no precise guidance about matters such as the quantity of bad things that one would be allowed to do to arrive at the good things. The answer that the pursuit of good must be limited to actions that do not produce bad things is too facile, given that human actions will usually produce some good and some bad. It is left to the individual to determine, or to a social group or a set of rituals (often of obscure origin) to indicate, what behavior is best under the circumstances.

Nor is it clear whose health and happiness, survival, knowledge, calmness, or knowledge should have priority. When it is impossible to satisfy everyone's ambitions, should the level of goodness be measured by the numbers of people who are receiving benefits—subtracting, for example, the number of people who will not receive benefits or whose benefits may have to be curtailed so that benefits can be provided to some? And how should the decision be reached when more than one good outcome could be pursued? Because many of the aims considered to be good (e.g., health) can only be reached if significant changes affecting everyone in a society are undertaken, it is also necessary to state how decisions about the course of action for other desirable goals will be made and enforced. How much coercion is acceptable for the common good? And acceptable to whom? How do we resolve the conflict between families', communities', and broader society's needs?

Faced with the variety of cultural and other differences across the world, and in the absence of external criteria and evidence that would help in the answering of questions like those just listed and allow the formulation of rules of behavior based on ethical principles confirmed by evidence, professionals of many disciplines decided to compose guidelines for ethical behavior by consensus. This decision is based on the belief that by incorporating the experience and opinions of many in a consensus about a course of action, we can make such a consensus closer to timeless and culture-free ethical paradigms. However, it is clear, though sometimes forgotten, that consensus and democratic decisions regarding matters about which we have no external (e.g., scientific) evidence are not necessarily the same as the truth. Each instance of nonconformism with consensus-based statements should therefore be considered carefully, because the nonconformist position might be more creative and more contributory to the good and thus require a reexamination of the consensus.

Once it is accepted that the rules of behavior agreed on by a worldwide consensus are the best possible substitute for the rules of ethical behavior of professionals based on timeless and cross-culturally valid paradigms of ideal behavior in a profession, it is necessary to examine whether the moral rules of behavior for the profession are, on the whole, close to these ethical rules. This exploration must cover rules for the performance of clinical duties, research, and teaching activities, but it cannot stop there. The behavior of psychiatrists in the public arena must also be explored, perhaps even more than the behavior of other professionals. The stigma and special position of psychiatry in society, for example, make it likely that unbecoming conduct will not only tarnish the particular psychiatrist's reputation but also affect the image of the profession as a whole, which in turn might slow the development of programs that could help patients, thus diminishing the usefulness of the profession as a whole.

The consensus among members of a profession, including psychiatry, is often based on consensus of representatives of political groups, national governments, and groups of international and national, nongovernmental and governmental organizations. For example, in 1948 the World Medical Association (WMA) produced the Declaration of Geneva, which states the duties of the person "being admitted as a member of the medical profession" (Bojadjiev 1996, p. 9). The text of the declaration is very similar to the Hippocratic Oath, although there are differences, mainly results of attempts to make the text acceptable to the majority of the delegates. Other differences are due to changes in society and culture over the many years since antiquity, when the ethical principles of professional conduct were produced. However, these changes are minor—an indication that what was proposed has a certain timelessness, which should be a mark of the truth.

The WMA produced a number of other consensus statements, including the International Code of Medical Ethics (1949; amended in 1968 and 1983) and the Declaration of Helsinki (1964), which concerns biomedical research involving human subjects. Many of the consensus statements of the WMA have been amended several times, exemplifying the need to examine whether the rules defined at a point in time remain applicable. These general statements have also been complemented by a series of others regarding the behavior of physicians in different situations—when functioning in a national health care system (1963), at times of armed conflict (1956), or in rural areas (1964) or when faced with the coercion to participate in torture (1975). Furthermore, the WMA also addressed the behavior of doctors in relation to therapeutic abortion (1970), family planning (1967), and the new challenges to confidentiality presented by the rapid spread of use of computers in medicine (1973). Over the years, the WMA has produced no fewer than 74 statements on the behavior of medical doctors in different situations and in the performance of tasks of the profession (Bojadjiev 1996). There is no doubt that the WMA will continue this tradition of amending statements or producing new ones.

In addition to the WMA, other agencies have also produced important statements by international consensus. Among these, two statement by the United Nations stand out: the Principles of Medical Ethics (UN Resolution 37/194) (Bankowski and Howard-Jones 1982) and the statement concerning the protection of persons with mental illness and the improvement of mental health care. The latter statement is of particular interest to psychiatrists because it indicates not only that mentally ill patients have the right not to be abused but also that they have "the right to the best available mental health care." The importance of this resolution (46/119, adopted by the General Assembly of the United Nations in 1991) is both theoretical and practical; in adopting this resolution, the United Nations, the world's supreme political body, has stated ethical principles that should govern the provision of care and has created the legal basis for the provision of mental health care, because receiving such care is a human right.

The World Psychiatric Association produced several statements about ethical behavior and the duties of psychiatrists. The first of these were the Declaration of Hawaii (amended in Vienna in 1983) and the World Psychiatric Association Statement and Viewpoints on the Rights and Legal Safeguards of the Mentally Ill (1989; cited in Bojadjiev 1996). In 1996, the World Psychiatric Association produced the Declaration of Madrid (see the Appendix to this book), an updated consensus statement on ethical issues and related to psychiatry, accompanied by a series of guidelines about the behavior of psychiatrists in specific situations (e.g., in relation to euthanasia).

These documents and resolutions deal with the practice of psychiatry and the behavior of psychiatrists in specific situations. The rules of ethical conduct of medical doctors in general (and of psychiatrists in particular) in relation to research have been discussed in a range of documents. A number of countries have passed legislation requiring that institutions financing or hosting research establish ethical committees and other mechanisms to ensure that research is conducted according to specific guidelines regarding experimentation and medical ethics. International organizations (e.g., the Council for International Organizations of Medical Sciences [Bankowski and Howard-Jones 1982]) have convened meetings of ethicists, health care decision-makers, and researchers to define minimal ethical standards for scientific investigations and have made recommendations (e.g., Council for International Organizations of Medical Sciences 1993; Howard-Jones and Bankowski 1979). Rules about research in general have been complemented by rules about epidemiological research (Bankowski et al. 1991) and other types of studies. Unfortunately, there are still many countries in which investigations can be undertaken without the explicit approval of an independent ethical committee. In some countries, ethical committees have been established (often because of pressure exerted by investigators whose proposals were not eligible for international support without the approval of such bodies) but are not independent and do no more than rubber-stamp proposals made by influential members of the academic community. Also, in some instances researchers from industrialized countries with significant research funding find ways to carry out research in a developing country in which ethical control is less strict. Funding agencies and editors of widely read and respected scientific journals are gradually requiring approval of an independent ethical committee before proceeding to fund a particular project or publish its results. Rules for ethical behavior, in relation to collaborators in international research, have been proposed because of the frequency of asymmetrical and often exploitative relations in a variety of countries and situations over the years (Sartorius 1988).

Although ethical aspects of research have become a standard part of the agenda of research funding agencies and relevant governmental and nongovernmental organizations, examination of ethical aspects of proposals for the purpose of reform of medical education or of restructuring medical or nursing curriculum is still rare, even though changes in medical education have a profound impact on the ethical behavior of whole generations of students and doctors. There is generally little or no pressure to present evidence to the government and to society that a particular reform will not only produce some gains in terms of knowledge and skills but also contribute to the development of the propensity to act in accordance with ethical principles.

Ethics and National
Mental Health Programs

In the 1960s and 1970s, it was sufficient to reach a consensus on a text such as the Declaration of Madrid, translate the text into many languages, recommend application of the principles to psychiatric societies, and insist that these principles be reflected in research training and practice of psychiatry. Today, not only are translation, distribution, and promotion required (many of the earlier important documents and guidelines were not handled this way), but other steps must be undertaken as well. These steps stem from the currently more and more widely used strategy of mental health program development.

This strategy was first introduced some 20 years ago (Sartorius 1978). It generally takes two decades (one working generation), if not more, for a strategy to become a self-evident way of proceeding (Sartorius 1982). The new mental health program development strategy has three main features. First, mental health programs must encompass more than the treatment of mental disorders and the rehabilitation of the mentally ill. Promotion of mental health—that is, a systematic effort to enhance the value assigned to mental health by individuals, communities, and societies—must become part of mental health programs. Without that element, it is unlikely that mental health programs will become part and parcel of overall health and social development programs and that the population will be willing to invest in the improvement of mental health, the care of the mentally ill, and other components of the program (Sartorius 1998). Prevention of mental diseases—possible at primary, secondary, and tertiary levels, as is the case with any other group of diseases—is an additional necessary component, one that is often lacking (Sartorius and Henderson 1992). Another often neglected task of mental health programs is to contribute to the reduction of psychosocial problems, such as violence and drug abuse, and to ensure that psychosocial aspects of medical practice in general receive the attention they deserve.

The second characteristic of the overall strategy for mental health programs is a logical consequence of the first. The multitude of tasks that need to be undertaken to make progress in the areas of work just described cannot be accomplished by psychiatrists alone. Other professions, governmental health sector and sectors not related to health, patient and family organizations, industry, and the community must all be actively involved in the development, implementation, and evaluation of mental health programs. The establishment of a permanent collaboration and communication among these partners ("The Pentalogue") is a particularly high priority for programs of the future (Sartorius 1999).

The third feature of the strategy for mental health programs concerns the strategy's temporal validity. In the past, it was possible to make plans for long periods because changes were unlikely to occur very quickly. Today, however, in addition to overall long-term goals, programs must have short-term plans that are sufficiently flexible to allow for changes because of increased knowledge and technological progress, socioeconomic change, or change in overall strategies of governments. "Rolling horizon" planning, in which there is constant evaluation and adjustment of work plans, requires a different structure of programs and a different attitude by staff, both difficult but possible to introduce.

All three of these features of mental health programs have an impact on the formulation and permanence of ethical guidelines for psychiatry. The ethical guidelines must cover psychiatrists' conduct in the performance of all of the duties in the expanded list of tasks. If psychiatrists are to help prevent mental illness, they must learn how to deal with the media, and the ethical codes must be formulated so that it is ensured that this relationship is ethically acceptable. If psychiatrists are to become involved in one way or another in the process of changing people's values, to promote mental health, there should be specific ethical guidelines that help them to remain on the correct path, avoiding conflict resulting from promotion of other, equally noble purposes. If psychiatrists are to be active in the programs that deal with the reduction of psychosocial problems, they must define—as a profession and by consensus—the limits of their action and how they will operate in areas in which scientific evidence is feeble and many factors are at work.

The second characteristic of the mental health program strategy also affects the formulation of ethical guidelines and deontological principles or statements. If it is true that psychiatrists cannot develop appropriate mental health programs alone—and there is ample evidence that this is the case— they will need to discuss the framework for their behavior and the ethical standards that they will accept with the other participants in the development of mental health programs: professional organizations, organizations of families and of patients, and representatives of relevant sectors of the government and of industry.

These discussions are unlikely to be calm and agreeable; the interests of the participants in the development of mental health programs are often opposed and hidden. Patients may wish to have the right to choose a treatment style (for example, treatment without the use of medicaments); governments, on the other hand, might be interested in keeping the cost of treatment down—by, for example, reducing the number of reimbursable treatment options. Governments might also wish to promote the use of the most cost-effective treatments, opposing physicians who might wish to choose treatments that are most beneficial for their patients, even if these treatments are not the most cost-effective. In a free-market economy, industry—the pharmaceutical industry and other industries involved in health care—seeks to maintain its profits, which might make purchase of the best treatment difficult for patients or their families. Families' interests are not always identical to those of patients. There is often no agreement within the profession or with the other groups concerned; in addition, patient and family organizations, industry, governmental sectors, and the professions across countries are far from agreement about the most desirable behavior or about other matters of relevance in this argument (e.g., what might constitute the best form of care).

The third feature of modern mental health programs also influences the formulation of desirable standards of ethical and moral behavior of psychiatrists and other mental health professionals. Long-term goals of mental health programs must be formulated in general terms; they will resemble ethical standards. Short-term goals, on the other hand, must be formulated with the situation in which the program is being implemented taken into account—thus in terms similar to those used in the description of the moral behavior of health care staff, which will always depend on the actual situation.

Future Action

From the considerations presented in this chapter, it is possible to make recommendations concerning future action. These recommendations are made in the belief that it is likely that our understanding of good and evil will continue to progress; that there are universally applicable paradigms of behavior of members of the medical profession that are based on the furtherance of good and diminution of evil; and that it is possible to define rules of behavior that will be congruent with these paradigms and help the medical professions, including psychiatry, to make a positive contribution to the good of individuals and society as a whole.

1. Ethicists must continue studying professional behavior, with the explicit goal of defining ideal standards of behavior for the profession, standards whose implementation will allow the determination of activities most likely to increase the total good for individuals and societies while avoid-

ing harm and bad consequences by the members of the profession and other involved in relevant programs.

2. Ethical behavior of members of the mental health professions should be promoted, and mental health professionals should act according to ethical standards of universal validity. In this respect, the following principles seem to be emerging and slowly gaining general acceptance:

  i. Those involved in mental health programs must respect all participants in the process and should in turn be respected by them. This means that psychiatrists must respect the interests and welfare of their patients while also respecting and examining the interests of all others involved in mental health care—from families and other caregivers to industry and the various sectors of government. In turn, these other participants in the process should respect the views and positions of psychiatrists and other mental health professionals.

  ii. The principle of avoiding or minimizing harm (i.e., suffering; loss of personal and family autonomy; and material, human, and moral damage) should have high priority in any action having the goal of increasing benefits for the patient, the family, and society. The other principles often quoted as being important in the ethical performance of medicine are less likely to be universally applicable at this point in time. The principle of autonomy of the individual is one example. In many cultures, interests and preservation of a social group (e.g., a family) take precedence over the interests and even survival of the individual. The principle of beneficence is widely accepted, but the definition of beneficence and the interpretation of the concept are likely to vary. The principle of equity in care provision is also less likely to be generalizable in the short run, because equity in health care can best be maintained when there is equity in society and most societies of the world are unfortunately far from reaching that goal. In light of this situation, psychiatrists should try to act in accordance with all four tenets of ethical behavior—remaining aware, however, that progress might be uneven and that the priority given to each of them might differ from society to society and from time to time.

  iii. In determining guidelines for ethical behavior, psychiatrists should take into account the views and recommendations of all participants in mental health programs. The process of reaching consensus concerning ethical guidelines for the practice of psychiatry as a discipline should be guided by available evidence and experience from as many settings as possible.

3. Psychiatrists practice in different countries and belong to different cultures. This might make their moral behavior different from that guided by universally promoted ethical standards. In these situations, psychiatrists should make every effort to act in accordance with universally accepted principles of ethical behavior and advocate the acceptance of these principles by other mental health professionals and by all other participants in mental health programs.

4. Given the imperfection of their understanding of good and bad and the likelihood that moral obligations in different societies will change over time, psychiatrists should ensure the regular reexamination of guidelines for the application of ethical principles in psychiatry and in mental health programs.

References

Bankowski Z, Howard-Jones N (eds): Human Experimentation and Medical Ethics. Geneva, Switzerland, Council for International Organizations of Medical Sciences, 1982

Bankowski Z, Bryant JH, Last JM (eds): Ethics and Epidemiology: International Guidelines. Geneva, Switzerland, Council for International Organizations of Medical Sciences, 1991

Bilimoria P: Indian ethics, in A Companion to Ethics. Edited by Singer P. Oxford, England, Blackwell, 1997, pp 43–58

Bojadjiev B: Physicians, Patients, Society, Human Rights and Professional Responsibilities of Physicians in Documents of International Organizations. Amsterdam, Kiev, Geneva Initiative, 1996

Council for International Organizations of Medical Sciences: International Ethical Guidelines for Biomedical Research Involving Human Subjects. Geneva, Switzerland, Council for International Organizations of Medical Sciences, 1993

Howard-Jones N, Bankowski Z (eds): Medical Experimentation and the Protection of Human Rights. Geneva, Switzerland, Council for International Organizations of Medical Sciences; Geneva, Switzerland, Sandoz Institute for Health and Socio-Economic Studies, 1979

Kuhn TS: The Structure of Scientific Revolutions. Chicago, IL, University of Chicago Press, 1970

Sartorius N: The new mental health programme of WHO. Interdisciplinary Science Reviews 3:202–206, 1978

Sartorius N: Epidemiology and mental health policy, in Public Mental Health. Edited by Wagenfeld MO, Lemkau PV, Justice B. Beverly Hills, CA, Sage, 1982, pp 131–142

Sartorius N: Experience from the mental health programme of the World Health Organization. Acta Psychiatr Scand Suppl 344:71–74, 1988

Sartorius N, Henderson AS: The neglect of prevention in psychiatry. Aust N Z J Psychiatry 26:550–553, 1992

Sartorius N: Universal strategies for the prevention of mental illness and the promotion of mental health, in Preventing Mental Illness: Mental Health Promotion in Primary Care. Edited by Jenkins R, Ustün TB. New York, Wiley, 1998, pp 61–67

Sartorius N: Social justice, responsibility, and solidarity. Keynote lecture presented at the XI World Congress of Psychiatry, Hamburg, Germany, August 6–11, 1999

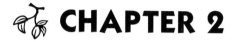 # CHAPTER 2

The Impact of Arab Culture on Psychiatric Ethics

Prof. Ahmed Okasha

Like most lads among my boyhood associates, I learned the Ten Commandments. I was taught to reverence them because I was assured that they came down from the skies into the hands of Moses, and that obedience to them was, therefore, secretly incumbent upon me. I remember that whenever I fibbed, I found consolation in the fact that there was no commandment, "Thou shalt not lie," and that the Decalogue forbade lying only as a "false witness" giving testimony before the courts where it might damage one's neighbor. In later years, when I was much older, I began to be troubled by the fact that a code of morals which did not forbid lying seemed imperfect; but it was a long time before I raised the interesting question: How has my own realization of this imperfection arisen? Where did I myself get the moral yardstick by which I discovered this shortcoming in the Decalogue? When that experience began, it was a dark day for my inherited respect for the theological dogma of "revelation." I had more disquieting experiences before me when, as a young orientalist, I found that the Egyptians had possessed a standard of morals far superior to that of the Decalogue over a thousand years before the Decalogue was written. (Breasted 1934, p. xi)

The quotation of Breasted is given here not to show that ethical guidelines and values originated from ancient Egypt but to show that the need for such codes dates back to ancient times. Since very early human interactions, relationships had to be regulated by means of ethical guidelines. Such codes are necessary to coordinate and control everyday interactions (These codes are generally laws.). The need for codes becomes more urgent when a hierarchy of power exists; the aim of these codes is to protect the less powerful from the control of the more powerful and to protect those with more power from claims of power abuse made by those with less power.

Since early in history, the doctor-patient relationship has been one of the major power relationships. In fact, doctors have been believed to have supernatural powers. Today, however, doctors are considered not half-gods but service providers whose primary tasks are to respond to the needs of their patients and to act in their patients' best interest. Furthermore, in the last 40 years there has been an advance in medical technology and knowledge, an advance that carries major hopes for the management of previously incurable ailments. However, there are also possibilities of abuse.

Psychiatry is one branch of medicine in which possibilities of abuse exist, and, indeed, actual abuse has occurred in this field. Because it involves investigation of the brain and its sometimes obscure functions, psychiatry has a mystique that not only is perceived by laypeople but may lead the psychiatrist to have a false sense of omnipotence. Mental illness remains an obscure, frightening type of illness because it frequently affects an important human attribute, judgment. A situation in which a patient has distorted judgment can be a good opportunity for abuse by any of several power structures—political, industrial, administrative, or even familial.

It is no wonder, therefore, that psychiatric associations all over the world have been trying hard to develop ethical codes with aims of protecting patients from possible abuse by members of the profession and preventing psychiatrists from feeling omnipotent.

The Declaration of Madrid

The Declaration of Hawaii issued by the World Psychiatric Association in 1977 led to a long process of investigation and to concern within the domain of professional ethics; it also paved the way for the Declaration of Madrid (see the Appendix to this book), which was endorsed by the General Assembly of the World Psychiatric Association in Madrid in 1996. In its final form, the Declaration of Madrid includes seven general guidelines that focus on the aims of psychiatry—namely, to treat mentally ill patients, prevent mental illness, promote mental health, and provide care and rehabilitation to mentally ill patients. The declaration prohibits abuse and prohibits the provision of treatment against a patient's will unless such treatment is necessary for the welfare and safety of the patient and others. Emphasis is placed on advising the patient or caregiver of all details of management and informing him or her about confidentiality and the ethics of research. An appendix to the declaration includes guidelines on specific ethical issues in psychiatry (i.e., euthanasia, torture, the death penalty, sex selection, and organ transplantation) as well as a summary of the 1991 United Nations resolutions on the rights of patients with mental illness. Further ethical guidelines were endorsed by the General Assembly of the World Psychiatric Association in Hamburg in August 1999—namely, regarding genetic research and counseling, discrimination on ethnic or cultural grounds, and psychiatrists addressing the media. Specific issues currently in preparation by the Ethics Committee of the World Psychiatric Association are the ethics of psychotherapy, the relationship of psychiatry with industry, the ethics of managed care, and the abuse of psychiatrists by third parties (e.g., managed care, insurance companies). Issues of patient consent and autonomy are addressed in the Declaration of Madrid, and absolute commitment to patient welfare and condemnation of abuse by political institutions or other parties are evident in the declaration and its appendices.

Universality of Human Rights Declarations

Unfortunately, the development of declarations is not the end of the story. In human rights conventions all over the world, there is the assumption that a social and political setup is present in which the individual being is the center of social attention. In the Declaration of Madrid, as in other declarations, it is assumed that a social setup is present in which the individual is the focus and in charge. What if this is not the case everywhere in the world?

Although it is true that the more international input there is in the drafting of a declaration, the more likely it is that all difficulties will be considered in the declaration, in the end a document is needed in which the major principles are highlighted. We believe that implementation of codes of ethics is frequently difficult because of the cultural and social setups in which the attempts at implementation are being made. These difficulties stem not only from interactions between individuals, families, and the community but also from the social position of the medical doctor and the hierarchical structure of the medical profession vis-à-vis the rest of the community. Religion and other beliefs also have an effect on the lives and behavior of people.

Malpractice is one of the main targets of ethical codes; an aim of such codes is to outline, address, and prevent malpractice. In the Arab region, malpractice does exist, but the reaction of people to malpractice is not the same as in many other regions of the world. For example, it is very rare for people in the Arab world to sue their doctors. This is due not only to the belief that whatever the doctor decides is the right thing but also to the conviction that the final outcome is determined by God alone. This judicial relationship with God almost saves people any responsibility for the outcome of medical interventions. This is even more the case with illnesses of an ambiguous nature, and most particularly psychiatric disorders.

Cultural Specificity

In Arab culture, the humanitarian interaction with a doctor is valued as much, if not more, than his or her technical ability or scientific knowledge. The humanitarian nature of this interaction depends on the way the doctor deals with the patient and his or her family and the extent to which the doctor expresses respect for and acceptance of local cultural and spiritual norms.

These norms may face us sometimes with questions such as the following: Do patients who are not told the diagnosis usually know it anyway? Is this information later communicated by verbal or nonverbal means? Is the interaction between patient and family different when the patient is the head of the household?

In Eastern cultures, social integration is emphasized more than autonomy; that is, the family, not the individual, is the unit of society. Dependence is more natural and infirmity is less alien in these cultures. When affiliation is more important than achievement, how one appears to others becomes vital and shame, rather than guilt, becomes a driving force. In the same manner, physical illness and somatic manifestations of psychological distress become more understood and acceptable and evoke a caring response; in contrast, a vague complaint of psychological symptoms may be disregarded or be considered to indicate that the patient is "soft" or, worse, "insane."

In some cultures, and we argue that Arab culture is one of them, the collectivity of the community is valued rather than the individuality of its members. Decisions are made not at an individual level but at a familial, tribal, or communal level, in the best perceived collective interest. How can we adhere to our ethical guidelines and at the same time not disregard the local values and norms of our target population? How can we practice without showing disrespect or disregard for local values? On the other hand, how can we ensure that respect for the local culture does not become a pretext for bypassing ethical guidelines, to the detriment of our patients' rights?

Whether we like it or not, the encounters between psychiatry and law keep bringing us back to our conflicting conceptions of the value of health on the one hand and the value of liberty, integrity, and autonomy on the other. Cultural, ethnic, and sometimes sociodemographic data such as level of education, age, and gender suggest different attitudes regarding patient autonomy and informed consent. What is the perceived harm when members of the medical community violate cultural conventions and insist on telling the truth to patients? What are the disruptions of coping mechanisms of individuals and families? In what ways does acculturation change the beliefs of patients of various ethnicities?

To answer those questions, it may be helpful to consider how individuals interact in Arab culture. We may then be able to understand the challenges and difficulties involved in implementing guidelines such as the Declaration of Madrid.

One must first be familiar with the main characteristics that differentiate the position of the individual within his or her community in a traditional society from that in a Western society. Although societies should not to be considered stereotypically, general common attitudes can be assumed (Leff 1988).

Differences between the two types of societies are listed in Table 2–1. These differences are the mainstream norm and not an absolute description of a stereotyped behavior. Table 2–1 shows that cultural diversity may influence the implementation of ethics in different societies. In traditional societies, the family is an extended one, decision making is group and family oriented, and the Western attitude regarding individual autonomy does not exist. The concept of external control, dependence on God with regard to health and disease, and attribution of illness and recovery to God's will all maintain a healthy doctor-patient relationship, which makes trust, confidence, and compliance characteristic in traditional societies.

Arab culture includes traditional beliefs in devils, *jinn*, the evil eye, and so on (delusional cultural beliefs). The family structure is characterized by affiliated behavior at the expense of differentiating behavior. Also, rearing is oriented toward accommodation, conformity, cooperation, affection, and interdependence as opposed to individuation, intellectualization, independence, and compartmentalization. The extended family helps in managing intergenerational conflicts. Young individuals vacillate between two worlds, one following the values of Western societies and the other following the values and beliefs of traditional societies.

Another point worth mentioning is that the phenomenon of homeless mentally ill patients, common in the United States and Europe (especially af-

TABLE 2–1.   Differences between traditional and Western societies
regarding relationships and medical treatment

Traditional societies	Western societies
Family and group oriented	Individual oriented
Extended family (less geographical than previously, but conceptual)	Nuclear family
Status determined by age, position in family, and care of elderly	Status achieved by own efforts
Relationship between kin obligatory	Relationship between kin a matter of individual choice
Arranged marriage, with an element of choice dependent on interfamilial relationship	Choice of marital partner; determined by interpersonal relationship
Extensive knowledge about distant relatives' lives	Knowledge about close relatives' lives only
Family decision-making	Individual autonomy
External locus of control	Internal locus of control
Physician's decision respected and considered holy	Doubt in doctor-patient relationship
Rare suing for malpractice	Common suing for malpractice
Deference to God's will	Self-determination
Healthy doctor-patient relationship	Mistrust in doctor-patient relationship
Individual can be replaced; family should continue and pride is in family tie	Individual is irreplaceable; pride is in self
Pride in family care of mentally ill patient	Community care of mentally ill patient
Dependence on God regarding health and disease; illness and recovery attributed to God	Self-determined recovery

ter mental health reform and the closing of psychiatric hospitals), is rare in
the Arab world. When it does occur, it is because of poverty and not because
of mental illness. Families in some traditional societies take pride in looking
after their mentally ill relatives. In these societies, it is shameful to the family
if it is discovered that a mentally ill family member is homeless.

Traditional Versus Modern Healing

There are a number of important lessons to be learned from the examination
of beliefs and practices relating to psychiatric illnesses that exist in various

cultures throughout the world. In many non-Western cultures, native practitioners, to whom modern psychiatry is completely unknown, treat emotionally disturbed persons. Examination of the emotional attitude and interpersonal elements in these various forms of psychological treatments gives the psychiatrist a broad perspective from which to study the basic components of present-day psychiatry and the ethics that guide it.

Traditional forms of mental health care contain important elements and are sometimes effective. Such treatments are frequently the only methods available in some cultures, a fact that requires better understanding to clarify the complex ways in which mental illness interacts with culture. Traditional treatments are characterized as culturally compatible (healers are familiar with the cultural value systems of the patients) and holistic (physical, psychological, social, and spiritual aspects of healing are integrated) and are usually carried out by charismatic healers—individuals who promise to be in charge and indeed are, almost to the point of bearing the responsibility for the results of their decisions. The therapeutic process also frequently incorporates the family, tribe, or group and involves the social manipulation of the patient's immediate environment.

Traditional and religious healers in primary psychiatric care deal with minor neurotic, psychosomatic, and transient psychotic states using religious and group therapies (e.g., the Zar ceremony), suggestion, devices, amulets, and incantations. National health priorities and health care services are not geared toward mental health and mentally ill patients. Furthermore, 75%–80% of Egyptian psychiatric patients, for example, present with somatic symptoms, and 60%–70% of these patients with somatic symptoms present to traditional healers and general practitioners (Okasha and Karam 1998).

In Arab culture, the patient's learning the diagnosis, prognosis, and lines of treatment is not viewed as empowering. In traditional societies, the family-centered model is valued. A higher value may be placed on harmonious functioning and the family rather than on autonomy of the individual family member.

The Role of Religion

Religion plays an important role in symptom phenomenology, attribution (God's will), and management. Psychological symptoms are attributed to weakness of personality, lack of faith, lack of conformity, laziness, or other factors, hardly factors that entitle an individual to a right of choice. Statements such as "if God is willing," "I seek refuge in God from the accursed Satan," "God is the healer" are widespread in the Arab world, indicating a belief that the final decision is made where no human has control and, therefore, that human choice is a marginal variable in the determination of the final outcome.

Islam is the religion of the majority in the Arab region. Fundamental in Islam is the essentially theocratic society, in which the state is of value only as the servant of revealed religion. This principle is explicitly stated in the constitutions of Morocco, Tunisia, Syria, Mauritania, Sudan, Egypt, and Yemen (David and Brierly 1985).

The Arabic word *majnoun* ("insane") appears five times in the Koran; however, there it alludes not to insanity but rather to how people perceived prophets when they first attempted to guide the people to enlightenment with beliefs not conforming with the traditions of their societies. During the dark ages of Islam, *majnoun* referred to possession by *jinn*, but the proper Arabic meaning of the word is that of a shield or barrier on the mind.

In Islamic jurisprudence, it is emphasized that criminal responsibility is to be attributed only to sane adults capable of good reasoning (Dols 1992). No responsibility is attributed to children, psychotic adults, or sleeping or stuporous persons. In Islam, the welfare and care of an individual with mental illness are clearly the responsibility of the family, and not of the society or state.

Muslim law, down to its finest details, is an integral part of the Islamic religion and to the revelation that it represents. Consequently, no authority in the world is qualified to change it. Not to obey Muslim law is a sin leading to punishment as a heretic and, thereby, excludes one from the community of Islam.

In Mediterranean countries, many people—especially those living in Islamic societies—have an external locus of control and all events are considered God's will. Islam is centered on the idea of humans' obligation or duties rather than on any rights they may have. In that context, issues such as consent, autonomy, and decision making become complex matters.

In addition to the concept that the mentally ill individual is possessed, there is the concept that a person with mental illness is one who dares to be innovative, original, or creative or attempts to find alternatives to a static and stagnant mode of living. This concept is evident in attitudes toward certain mystics. For example, the expansion of self and consciousness in Sufism has been taken as a rationale to label some Sufis as psychotic. The autobiographies of some Sufis reveal the occurrence of psychotic symptoms and many mental sufferings in their paths to self-salvation (M. Rakhawy, personal communication, August 1989).

The third concept is that mental illness is the consequence of disharmony or constriction of consciousness, to which nonbelievers are susceptible. It is related to denaturing of one's basic structure (Al Fitrah) and disruption of harmonious existence by egoism, detachment, or alienation, partly due to loss of integrative insight.

Which concept of mental illness prevails in the Islamic world depends on whether development or deterioration of genuine Islamic issues is occurring. For instance, during deterioration, the concept that the mentally ill individual is possessed by evil spirits dominates, whereas during periods of enlightenment and creative epochs, the disharmony concept dominates.

In Islam, the unity of body and psyche is also recognized. The psyche (Elnafs) is mentioned 185 times in the Koran, with the word referring variously to the body, behavior, affect, and conduct.

The teaching of the great clinician Rhazes had a profound influence on Arab as well as European medicine. The two most important books of Rhazes are El Mansuri and Al-Hawi. The first work includes the definition and nature of temperaments and is the predominant comprehensive guide to physiognomy. Al-Hawi is considered the greatest medical encyclopedia produced by a Muslim physician. Translated into Latin in 1279 and published in 1486, it was the first clinical book that presented complaints, signs, and differential diagnoses of and effective treatments for illness. Avicenna's "El-Canoon" was published 100 years later and is a monumental educational and scientific book with better classification.

It is believed that the first Islamic hospital was established by the early ninth century in Baghdad and was modeled on Eastern Christian institutions, apparently mainly monastic infirmaries. Of the hospitals that appeared throughout the Islamic world, perhaps the most famous was that created in Cairo by the Egyptian sultan al-Mansour Kalaoon in 1284 (Dols 1992).

The first psychiatric hospital in Europe was established in Spain, in the medieval Moorish kingdom of Granada, through Arab influence.

The fourteenth-century Kalaoon Hospital in Cairo had sections for surgery, ophthalmology, and treatment of medical and mental illnesses. Contributions by wealthy residents of Cairo made possible a high standard of medical care and periods of convalescence for patients until they could be gainfully employed. The care of mentally ill patients in a general hospital and the involvement of the community in the welfare of patients foreshadowed modern trends by six centuries (Baasher 1975).

Consent

The primary purpose of highlighting consent as a core element in psychiatric ethics is to promote individual autonomy and to permit rational decision-making. Consent is not the mere signing of a piece of paper by a patient to protect the treating physician or institution from future malpractice complaints. The risks and benefits of the proposed treatment and alternative treatments should be explained to the patient. Also, the patient should be informed about the risks and benefits of refusal of treatment, and it should be determined that the patient is not under any sort of undue influence and that the environment is not coercive. The basic elements of informed consent are competence (this involves the capacity for decision making; affective incompetence is not usually recognized by the law), information (there should be a fiduciary relationship in which there is respect for the dignity and autonomy of the patient), and noncoercion (there is a subtle difference between coercion and persuasion).

In common law, consent is not required in cases of necessity—when the doctor is of the opinion that treatment is in the patient's best interest and the patient is not competent to give valid consent to that treatment—and in emergency situations—when treatment is required in order to prevent immediate serious harm to a patient or to others.

Competence

Patients are considered legally competent unless legally judged incompetent or temporarily incapacitated by a medical emergency. In a 1948 ruling, the civil court held that persons are competent to make treatment decisions if they are of "sufficient mind to reasonably understand the conditions, the nature and the effect of the proposed treatment, [and the] attendant risks in pursuing the treatment and in not pursuing the treatment" (Egyptian Civil Law 1948, p. 44).

Common law states that competent adults have a right to refuse medical treatment even if refusal may result in death or permanent injury. Furthermore, competence can apply to different things; one may be competent to consent to treatment, to admit oneself to a hospital, or to agree to a "do not resuscitate" order.

Decision Making

What if the decision-making process is not an individual one? In Arab culture, issues of illness are dealt with as family matters. Whether a patient is hospitalized, for example, or subject to electroconvulsive therapy or discharged from the hospital is dependent not on what the patient wants himself or herself but on the estimation, need, or wish of the extended family. Patients may wish at times not to be burdened with the extra load of making decisions that may determine the patterns of the rest of their lives. The concept of shared responsibility is central in Arab culture, and most people in the Arab world would not like to be responsible for the outcomes of decisions made on their own.

The decision-making style in Arab culture might be best described as family centered. The moral, social, and psychological support for which extended families in developing countries are so well known is the result of collectivity of decision making, that is, decision making by consensus. An individual decision that differs from the collective decision leaves the decision maker to bear the responsibility of the outcome alone and may deprive him or her of familial support. On the other hand, when a collective decision is acted on, negative consequences of the decision are not the patient's fault alone and he or she does not have to bear the guilt of making a wrong decision.

One illustrative example of the issue of consent and decision making is hospital admission. In the United States, 73% of patients in psychiatric facilities are voluntarily admitted, whereas in Egypt, the rate is 90%. In reality, the distinction between voluntary and involuntary admission is not as clear as is stated in law. Patients are often pressured into agreeing to voluntary admission. If voluntary admission were always strictly voluntary, the rate of involuntary admission would likely increase. The family plays a strong role in the rate of voluntary admission. In the Arab world, respect for and compliance with family decisions is more important than autonomy of the individual, especially if responsibility for the outpatient rests with the family because there are no community social support systems.

It is the responsibility of the family to learn the patient's diagnosis and prognosis and to make the difficult decisions needed. Studies in Italy, Greece, Spain, and Egypt showed that a patient's learning of his or her diagnosis of cancer is not viewed as empowering. Rather, this knowledge is seen as isolating and burdensome to the patient, who is suffering too much and is too ignorant about his or her condition to be able to make meaningful choices. Knowledge of a diagnosis harms the patient by causing him or her to lose hope.

Affiliation Versus Autonomy

The idea of patient autonomy is not universal, nor has the level of patient autonomy remained constant. In 1961, 90% of physicians in the United States did not inform their patients of a diagnosis of cancer (Blackhall et al. 1995). In 1979, however, 97% of American physicians made it their policy to inform patients with cancer of their diagnosis. In most of the literature on this change, the view is that this is the result of the progress from physician paternalism, in which the patient remains uninformed, to a more enlightened and respectful attitude toward the patient.

The same change has occurred in the area of mental illness in some parts of the world. Cultural, ethnic, and probably sociodemographic factors affect attitudes regarding patient autonomy and informed consent.

In family-centered cultures, a higher value may be placed on the harmonious functioning of the family than on the autonomy of individual family members. Although it is true that the patient-autonomy model is founded on the idea of respect for persons, people live, become ill, and die in the context of family and culture and exist not simply as individuals but in a web of relationships (Blackhall et al. 1995).

Insisting on the patient-autonomy model of medical decision-making when that model runs counter to the deepest values of the patient may be another form of physician paternalism. In the Arab region, a person may actually change doctors because of the way the first doctor conveys information to him or her or if the doctor persists in considering the patient the only decision maker.

Confidentiality

A third major element of psychiatric ethics is confidentiality and disclosure of information, another universal principle of the Declaration of Madrid and other professional declarations. Although there is no consistently accepted set of information to be disclosed for any given medical or psychiatric situation, five pieces of information are generally provided: diagnosis; nature and purpose of the proposed treatment; consequences, risks, and benefits of the proposed treatment; viable alternatives to the proposed treatment; and prognosis (projected outcomes of treatment and no treatment).

Nurses, residents, social workers, psychologists, medical secretaries, insurance companies, and accreditation bodies already have access to this information and are entitled to see the patient's records. The issue of confidentiality therefore relates to people outside the medical profession and its accessories—the patient's family, for example.

Telling the patient the truth about his or her condition, especially when the prognosis is poor or a major decision should be made, is not considered a virtue in Arab culture. In fact, although Arab families praise the technological advances of Western medicine, they always comment about the harshness of Western doctors, who tell their patients the truth regardless of the associated emotional trauma to the patient. In Arab culture, the norm is to convey the information to the family first and then leave it up almost entirely to the family to decide whether to inform the patient.

Frequently, an Arab family will speak of a cousin who "feels" that he or she may have cancer and who does not really want to know for sure. There is a strong conviction among Arab patients that not knowing the truth allows the patient to have the hope that things may become better. Issues such as writing a will or making other economic arrangements are hardly matters of concern, probably because Islamic law leaves little room for interference by the patient in such practical matters. Preparation for death, too, is not of great concern, because it is mainly a spiritual matter, with few practical implications. In the field of psychiatry, an Arab patient and his or her family always like to hear that the patient's condition will improve. The patient and the patient's family would rather see a psychiatrist who will insist that things will get better—even if the condition does not in fact improve or improves only for short periods—than a psychiatrist who will relate the outcome in statistical, scientific terms. Arabs tend to believe that recovery is God's will and lack of recovery may be due to failure on the part of the doctor.

Conclusions

An ethical foundation is necessary in psychiatric practice so that patients are not left at the mercy of the good intent of the practitioner. However, ethical codes must be implemented with tact and understanding of local constraints so that the image of the psychiatrist and psychiatry is not further jeopardized. We could, for example, suggest that physicians ask patients whether they wish to be informed about their illnesses and be involved in making decisions about their care or whether they prefer that their families be informed and handle such matters. In any case, the patient's wishes should be respected and the patient should be allowed to choose a family-centered decision-making style. In permitting this form of decision making, we are not abandoning our commitment to individual autonomy or its legal expression in informed consent. Rather, we are broadening our view of autonomy so that respect for persons includes respect for the cultural values they bring with them to the decision-making process.

References

Baasher T: The Arab countries, in World History of Psychiatry. Edited by Howels TG. New York, Churchill Livingstone, 1975, pp 97–123

Blackhall L, Murphy S, Frank G, et al: Ethnicity and attitudes toward patient autonomy. JAMA 274:820–825, 1995

Breasted JH: The Dawn of Conscience. New York, Scribner's, 1934

David R, Brierly J: Major Legal Systems in the World Today. London, Stevens, 1985

Dols MW: Majnun: The Madman in Medieval Islamic Society. Edited by Immisch DE. Oxford, Clarendon, 1992

Egyptian Civil Law: Article 45,46, Vol 131, p 44. Egyptian Official Documents. Cairo, Ameria Press, 1948

Leff J: Psychiatry Around the Globe: A Transcultural View (Gaskell Psychiatry Series). London, Royal College of Psychiatrists, 1988, p 79

Okasha A, Karam E: Mental health services and research in the Arab world. Acta Psychiatr Scand 98:406–413, 1998

Declaration of Hawaii. World Psychiatric Association, 1977

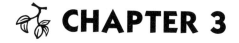

CHAPTER 3

Conflicts and Crises in Latin America

Prof. Julio Arboleda-Flórez
Prof. David N. Weisstub

To write on the sociological, legal, religious, ethical, or cultural aspects of the lives of a large number of people from different countries and ethnic and cultural backgrounds is a daunting task. There is a risk of making generalizations that do no justice to the peculiarities and idiosyncrasies of each group or country. Cultural characteristics and ethical values may vary from country to country and even from region to region.

Latin America comprises about 20 countries and extends roughly from the Rio Grande to Patagonia. Historians and geographers sometimes also include island states in the Caribbean. Altogether, Caribbean countries included, the region has about 480 million people, and the population is projected to be 810 million in 2050 (Bongaarts 1998). The main official languages in these countries are Spanish and Portuguese, but French, Dutch, and Creole are officially spoken in some of the Caribbean countries, and native languages are also recognized in some Central and South American countries. The main two languages, Spanish and Portuguese, and the predominant religion, Catholicism, reflect the Iberian heritage of these countries. Yet using the most obvious characteristics—heritage, language, and religion— to describe Latin America is a simplistic approach. Each country is host to many ethnicities, and the true characteristic of each country is the heterogeneity of the populations. Inhabitants in most of these countries have European ancestors. Yet indigenous populations—those peoples who inhabited the Americas before European settlers arrived in 1492—could be considered nations unto themselves. Different as well are the African descendants who make up large portions of the population in several of these countries.

Still, the three characteristics mentioned—heritage, language, and religion, reflections of European settlement—form the bases for the legal system and the institutional traditions in these countries. In turn, although culture, folklore, and beliefs about health and illness may vary from country to country, general characteristics can be discerned. Further, the ethical discourse in the region is very much based, with possible minor local variations, on Judeo-Christian (mostly Catholic) beliefs and values. Finally, the management of mentally ill patients in all of these countries reflects the styles and periods of reform in North America and Europe.

Culture and Conception of Illness

Several social and cultural factors in Latin American societies play roles in how inhabitants of the region regard health and illness and go about seeking help for their medical problems. The environment, religion, family attachments and values, gender, and sociopolitical changes all shape health-seeking behaviors.

Opler and Rennie (1956) pointed out: "Beginning with Kraepelin, it has been known that psychopathological illness varies in content and in type with culture" (p. 17). A society exists when many persons interact regularly and continuously on the basis of shared values and behaviors whose meanings have been previously established (Merrill 1961). The limits of a society are those of social interaction, which itself is essentially a process whereby two or more human beings take each other into account (Swanson 1965). Not only are culture, social systems, and personality functional variables; they are also interdependent and interrelated. Medical anthropology studies have shown that within the context of social interactions, the interdependence of these three variables permits people in different cultures and social groups to explain the causes of ill health, the types of treatment they believe in, and their choices of whom they turn to when they become ill. Members in a social group explain to themselves how these beliefs and practices relate to biological processes and psychological changes in the human organism in both health and illness (Helman 1994). Similarly, cultural explanations and beliefs regarding health and illness tend to be more holistic than technobiomedical explanations, and the environment is taken more into account. In many alternative health care systems, in fact, health and healing are defined in ways that reduce distinctions between the health of individuals and the health of their environments (Hufford 1996). In this regard, the advances in medicine and our scientific understanding of illness have not erased Hippocratic teachings (Hippocrates 1988) that permeate many cultural health-related beliefs in Latin America. A strong belief in an ecological understanding (Lolas 1986) of health and illness, coexisting with the medical model, is extensive in Latin America. Air, water quality, food, and timing of food intake are considered to have effects on illness and recovery.

Family values and closely knit communities play important roles in how health and illness are defined in Latin America. Family values hold the person to the group and help in curbing individual behavior. They place limits and impose duties on the individual. In Latin America, the family includes not only the nuclear family—parents and children—but also the extended family—grandparents, aunts, uncles, nieces, nephews, grandchildren, and godparents and their families. A godparent, who is usually not a member of the immediate family, represents or stands on behalf of a parent at the moment that parent's child is baptized. The godparent must protect the child and provide an example to the child as he or she grows into adulthood. Godparents are surrogate parents. An element of the relationship between the godparent and child is the bond that develops. The parental duties of godparents and the bonds that develop extend and reinforce family ties. Godparents become full members of the family.

Although rigid adherence to traditional and ancestral hierarchies, or deferring to the eldest in family decision making, is not the norm in Latin America, individual actions are still shaped by group pressure and moral suasion. Maintaining strong traditional family ties and providing support are lifelong expectations. Not paying attention to these duties is a sign of bad faith, leading to reprobation and opprobrium. Members of the family have pride and should abide by the accepted mores of respect and dignity. These family traditions may have an impact on health-seeking behaviors, especially if by seeking help, secrets that bring harm on the family are revealed, as happens with teen pregnancy or when the black sheep of the family ends up in prison. Health-seeking behaviors are, then, determined by interplay between the individual, the immediate family group, and the social beliefs regarding the determinants of and the best treatment for the illness.

Religious attitudes and beliefs impart a sense of belonging and acceptance. The individual copes with illness, death, and other calamities by drawing strength and support from a supreme being whose will is not disputed, whose beneficence is expected and taken for granted, or whose wrath is feared. Hope and faith, as expressions of religious attitudes, are deeply entrenched in the belief system of Latin Americans. However, in science, these issues are considered peripheral or ignored altogether, out of blindness or out of frustration at not being able to measure them or to conceptualize them in scientific terms. Scientific constructs based on rationality and uniformity of natural laws do not leave much room for their expression. Yet a lack of scientific grasp should not lead to denial of their existence; hope and faith constitute the je ne sais quoi that is vital to recovery. In fact, it is because of the effect of hope and faith on recovery that we need double-blind studies and that we try to control the placebo effect in our experiments. It is hope that keeps chronically ill patients believing in a cure, scientific or miraculous, and it is faith that gives them the strength to overcome adversity. As Seguin (1986) wrote: "We negate faith in the name of rationality, and yet, we could not do this unless we had faith in rationality" (p. 129) (our translation).

In Latin America, religious beliefs and attitudes permeate the way disease—defined as a structural or physiological deviation from the norm—is reinterpreted from the scientific discourse of the physician into a culture of acceptance of the illness—defined as the personal sense of being ill. Faith makes the patient accept the suffering with resignation; hope instills a sense that the cure is based not so much on the healer and the treatment prescribed but on the will of the Creator.

Machismo, or the role assigned to men in Latin American culture, means that the man is the provider, the person responsible for the welfare of the family, the protector, and, most important, the person responsible for the honor of the family (Canino and Canino 1993). The culture of *machismo* has two impacts. First, men usually work outside the home to provide for family needs and women remain at home to tend the children, look after their husbands, and provide emotional support. The role of the man is to deal with the world outside, whereas the role of the woman is to cement the family ties from within the home. A loss of the provider role, or a reversal of roles, when the man cannot work because of unemployment or illness and the woman must work outside the home, causes the man to lose value among other men and may lead him to alcoholism. Latin American men tend to drown their pain through drinking, whereas women in Latin America tend to sit at home and cry.

The second impact of *machismo* relates to honor. *Machismo* imposes a duty on men not to back down in the face of an insult to the honor of a family member. Backing down brings shame not only to the man but to the whole family. To be *macho* means to be tough and to die or to kill for honor. Because of *machismo*, Latin American men try not to appear ill or they seek help only when it is absolutely necessary.

Finally, major sociopolitical upheavals and financial crises that have brought or threaten to bring radical change to the political structures in many countries in Latin America have affected cultural attitudes toward health and illness in the region. Rapid urbanization, many times resulting from guerrilla activity in the countryside, has led to social disorganization and lack of cohesion. Family units have been broken down and, in large cities, children are often abandoned. In many countries these upheavals include a veritable epidemic of violent behavior.

Psychiatry and Folk Illnesses

There are medical conditions that are peculiar to particular social groups or countries and do not have immediate biomedical explanations. These medical conditions are illnesses without disease and fall into the general category of folk illnesses. Rubel (1977) defined them as "syndromes from which members of a particular group claim to suffer and for which their culture provides an etiology, a diagnosis, preventive measures and regimens of healing" (p. 120). Folk illnesses are more than clusters of symptoms and physical signs. They have symbolic meaning—moral, social, or psychological—for the individuals with the illnesses. In folk illnesses, the suffering is linked to changes in the environment or the working of supernatural forces, and these illnesses signal, in a standardized, culturally acceptable way, social conflict or disharmony at home, with friends, or at work (Helman 1994). Mezzich and Lewis-Fernández (1997) emphasized the importance of understanding these links. These authors advised development of a cultural formulation that would take into account, among other things, the cultural identity of the individual and the cultural explanations of the illness.

In Latin America, cultural beliefs and popular conceptions of illness and health not only relate to physical illness but also include a host of psychiatric symptoms and a peculiar understanding of psychiatric illness. A review of some major cultural and folkloric ways in which illness is conceptualized in Latin America will therefore be useful.

Susto or *espanto* (magical fright) occurs in individuals all over Latin America, regardless of ethnicity, is found in urban and rural areas, and affects males and females alike. *Susto* also occurs in Hispanics in California, Texas, Colorado, and New Mexico. It is a whole syndrome that includes various somatic and psychological symptoms attributed to a traumatic event. The core belief is that because of sudden fright or an unsettling experience, the immaterial part of the human being is separated from the body and wanders about.

The resulting "soul loss" produces restlessness at night, anxiety, depression, listlessness, lassitude, inability to carry out expected functions at work or at home, loss of appetite, and lack of interest in activities or personal decorum. The condition is related to social situations in which the individual cannot meet social expectations. *Susto* is a vehicle through which Latin Americans in peasant or urban groups manifest their reactions to self-perceived stressful situations. Kiev (1972) would classify *susto* as an anxiety reaction. The treatment for *susto* is based on the need to recapture the soul and return it to its rightful place within the owner.

The evil eye *(mal de ojo)*, which is not specific to Latin America, relates to the fear that others will envy one's possessions (Spooner 1970). A person possessing the evil eye can harm unintentionally or intentionally and either is a stranger or is a local person whose attitudes or appearance differs from that of the rest of the people. It is particularly important if the person stares rather than speaks. The evil eye may cause emotional distress or physical illness or make the individual prone to disease or injury. Those affected by the evil eye, especially children, fail to thrive and begin having one ailment or infection after another. The evil eye can be counteracted by distracting attention or with sympathetic magic (Underwood and Underwood 1981).

An attack of nerves *(ataque de nervios)* is a common condition that is found in many countries in Latin America and affects individuals regardless of class, ethnicity, or gender. The attacks usually have an acute onset, with shaking, paresthesia, numbness of the face, inability to move, heat sensation, a feeling of dread, and a feeling of the mind going blank. There is usually a gradual buildup of uneasiness about family or financial problems, until the whole attack takes place (De La Cancela et al. 1986).

Widows and spurned lovers sometimes die of *pena moral* (a broken heart). After experiencing a major loss, the individual closes the inner self to the outside world by not leaving the home or bedroom, not eating, and not communicating. The person slowly withers away as the desire to live disappears, and no amount of encouragement or pleading to snap out of it and start living again will bring the person back. *Pena moral* is the equivalent of deep bereavement ending in major depression.

Another important factor to consider is the way Latin Americans seek help when illness strikes a member of the family. Often a person uses two healing systems: the Western model, involving physicians, and the holistic alternative system, involving *curanderos* (healers). The patient goes to a physician and takes the prescribed medications and then goes to a *curandero* or uses a variety of herbs or other remedies. *Curanderismo* and ethnopharmacological practices are, therefore, part and parcel of the culture. Typically, the *curandero*, akin to a shaman, conducts a diagnostic interview that consists mostly of questions about the life circumstances of the patient, makes a formulation, and prescribes some behavioral change and herbs. *Curanderos* are often the first health workers patients go to when affected by *susto*, the evil eye, or other folk conditions. The importance of their role cannot be minimized, given that many of these conditions may mask serious physical or mental problems.

It may be assumed that beliefs about health and illness, folk illnesses, and limits on individuality eventually interfere with the scientific management of medical conditions. It is proposed, however, that for Latin Americans, these cultural norms permit a sense of ownership of the illness and of mastering of the healing process.

Violence as a Psychiatric Epidemic

Violence in Latin America, as previously mentioned, has attained epidemic proportions. External causes, usually accidents and interpersonal violence, are among the most frequent causes of death in many countries of Latin America. Among individuals ages 15–24 years, accidents are the number one cause of death in all Latin American countries with more than one million people, except Colombia, and among persons ages 25–44 years, accidents are the number one cause among men and in the total population in all countries. Thus, whereas in Canada and United States only about 5% of all deaths are due to external causes, in Brazil and Mexico that rate is about 12%, and in Colombia and El Salvador it is about 25%. In Colombia and El Salvador, homicide is the most frequent external cause of death, much more frequent than motor vehicle accidents or any other kind of accident. Among men, whereas homicide is the fifth leading cause of death in Canada and the United States, in Guatemala it is the most frequent cause of death, and it is the second leading cause in Ecuador, Mexico, Brazil, El Salvador, Venezuela, Paraguay, Panama, and other countries (Pan American Health Organization 1990).

Possibly related to the religious heritage and the Catholic injunction against suicide, violence against the self is not common in Latin America compared with other countries, but the rate of homicide is much higher than in North America or Europe. For example, whereas in 1988 the rates for homicide and suicide were 1.3 and 10.6 per 100,000, respectively, in Canada and 7.5 and 8.9 per 100,000, respectively, in the United States, these rates were, respectively, 29.7 and 3.4 per 100,000 in Colombia, 41.6 and 12.2 per 100,000 in El Salvador, 13.3 and 2.8 per 100,000 in Brazil, and 19.6 and 2.1 per 100,000 in Mexico (Pan American Health Organization 1990). Clearly, Latin Americans do not kill themselves—they kill each other.

Large areas in many countries, and practically every major city, are no-man's-lands into which people venture at their peril. Countries such as Colombia, Mexico, and countries in Central America have been the most affected, and the morgues in some cities, such as São Paulo and Caracas are well used. For example, the *Folha de São Paulo* (1998) indicated that on average, about 54 persons are murdered in São Paulo every week. In some countries, such as Colombia, practically everyone's life has been touched by the wave of violence. Everyone in Colombia seems to have lost close family members, other relatives, close friends, neighbors, or work associates. Massacres, rampant and wanton violence, and homicides have been occurring in the country for more than 30 years, the result of guerrilla warfare driven by political ideologies or economic warfare on the state incited by powerful drug lords. Poverty, inequalities, social exclusion, and social unrest are the most important reasons for violence in Colombia, not personal acts or terrorist manifestations (Guerrero 1998). The same can be said for many other countries in Central and South America.

The costs of violence on the general health system have been enormous (Minayo 1994). The costs of human suffering have not been estimated, nor has the social damage caused by displacement of thousands of people from the countryside to cities. In the cities, human and sanitary services are already inadequate. New phenomena are the abandonment of children and the abuse of street children, damaging to future generations. Far worse is the "disposal" of street children and undesirable children in the big cities. Cases of posttraumatic stress disorder have only begun to be tallied in Colombia and other Latin American countries. The toll of lost lives and the potential years of life lost (especially among youths and young men in their potentially most economically productive stage), the social and economic costs, and the impacts on the already strained health services have made violence the number one health priority in Latin America. The cost of violence on social and health systems has already been recognized at the international level. The Pan American Health Organization (PAHO), the arm of the World Health Organization in the Americas, has taken action on the matter and has formulated a regional plan of action on violence and health. As part of the plan, PAHO convened, in Washington, the Inter-American Conference on Society, Violence and Health. At the conference, a declaration was issued that stated:

Violence constitutes a threat to peace, security and consolidation of democratic ideas in the Region of the Americas as it strains the social fabric and invites the adoption of repressive policies.

It is widespread and expresses itself in a multitude of ways.

It affects negatively quality of life, creates fear, destroys family structures, and curtails the autonomy of individuals.

It constitutes a growing problem for public health as demonstrated by the alarming increase of rates of mortality, morbidity, and disability, as well as in the overwhelming loss of potential years of life and psychological effects.

It exacts an enormous economic toll on society by generating growing expenditures on health and security.

It affects women in and out of the home. (Pan American Health Organization 1994)

It was presented at the conference that the origins of violence include such factors as inequality and social injustice that create frustration, marginalize populations, and perpetuate conflicts; that violence reflects a fragility of the social order; and that violence persists because of widespread impunity and government condonation. In the declaration, heads of state were requested to redouble their efforts to ensure people's safety and uphold the rule of law. People of the countries represented were urged to mobilize against violence, to report information on violence, to develop prevention and control mechanisms, to encourage the media and national organizations to support initiatives against violence by promoting a culture of peace, and to ask heads of state to adopt the principles of the declaration (Pan American Health Organization 1994). What effect this declaration and PAHO's initiatives will have on reducing violence in Latin America remains to be seen, but certainly countries in the region, nongovernmental organizations, and health care professionals, including psychiatrists, can no longer turn a blind eye to this reality.

Psychiatric Services

In many countries worldwide, epidemiological, family, and clinical studies point toward the high incidence of major depression in the general population and, specifically, among middle-aged women. The few reports from Latin America indicate that a similar situation exists in the region and that alcoholism and violence are problems mostly affecting men (Pan American Health Organization 1990). Yet with few exceptions (Organización Panamericana de la Salud 1995), epidemiological data are hard to come by that could permit planning of services based on population needs. On the other hand, historical, constitutional, financial, and sociopolitical factors have put pressure on the structure of psychiatric care and on the delivery of psychiatric services in Latin America over the past two decades.

With some exceptions, notably Colombia, Venezuela, Brazil, and Jamaica, countries in the region have been unable to rally behind a need to reform psychiatric services that have mostly been based on the model of the old psychiatric hospitals. Venezuela, for example, has a draft bill on mental health, protection, and care of mentally ill persons that would decentralize services and encourage community organization of systems while promoting patients' rights, the prevention of mental illness, and the maintenance of mental health in the population (División de Salud Mental 1993). Otherwise, most countries in the region are far behind in terms of mental health reform, which has occurred in Italy (Basaglia 1968), England (Hollingsworth 1996), Canada (Arboleda-Flórez and Copithorne 1994; Province of Ontario 1990), and the United States (Zeman and Schwartz 1994). The debates in Latin America about mental health services and the rights of mentally ill patients are distant echoes of what is already an accepted way of providing psychiatric services in many other countries (Ridgway 1997).

Responding to a cry for reform of outmoded structures and thinking patterns, representatives of 17 Latin American countries met in Caracas in 1990 to develop a consensus for the restructuring of psychiatric services in Latin America. A set of recommendations, now known as the Declaration of Caracas (González Uzcátegui and Levav 1991), was produced at this PAHO meeting. In the declaration, the parameters of services in the region were reviewed and guidelines for action were given.

Up to the time of the Declaration of Caracas (and even up to the present), psychiatric services in Latin America were institutionally based. As in many other regions, large psychiatric hospitals that were built at the end of the last century or the beginning of this century have seen better days. In many cases their physical structures have deteriorated and financial support, often entirely governmental, has seriously eroded. At the same time, dependence on psychiatric hospitals has brought the development of psychiatric thinking to a standstill. For example, although there are excellent research groups in some places, research is not common. Research includes a study of neurotransmitters by a group in São Paulo, a major epidemiological study of vulnerabilities and resilience among children in the shantytowns of Lima, a study of the social costs of mental illness in Mexico, and a major study of urban violence in Cali, Colombia.

There are also a poor distribution and a poor use of resources. In some countries, for example, psychiatrists and other mental health professionals dedicate much time and many resources to individual psychoanalytically based psychotherapy, but there are not enough human resources to otherwise treat the large number of mentally ill patients. Then, too, many other psychiatrists practice mostly in psychiatric hospitals and their private clinics and leave little time for work in the community. In many respects, mental health professionals have largely neglected the increasing number of sociobehavioral problems that are the result of poverty, overcrowding, socially stressful situations, and violence.

One important aspect of the Declaration of Caracas relates to the protection of the rights of mentally ill patients. Latin American countries lag behind in the developing of legislation in this area. It could be argued that considering patients' rights is a luxury and an exercise in byzantinism when entire populations are fighting for their own rights of free speech and for better economic conditions. Although most Latin American countries have moved away from military regimes and embraced democratic forms of government, multiple levels of discrimination prevent large sectors of the population from being accepted as full partners in the political process and into power structures in their own countries (Fox 1988). In this volatile social situation, political rights are the most immediate concern, and groups such as mentally ill patients that traditionally have been marginalized and disenfranchised receive far less attention. Thus sociopolitical problems and lack of government interest, public advocacy, and funds all play roles in keeping patients in decrepit and outmoded psychiatric institutions where protection of rights is possibly considered least important.

The fight to keep psychiatric hospitals going and protect the meager resources allocated to the treatment of patients with chronic mental illness has siphoned the energies of health care providers and patient advocates. When survival is the only concern, rights become a secondary issue or an unaffordable luxury. Yet keeping psychiatric hospitals running has also had a more pernicious effect on the development of alternative forms of treatment. The inertia and isolation brought about by working in psychiatric hospitals, away from the hustle and bustle of general hospital psychiatry, outpatient activities, and community involvement, have meant that few resources are diverted to the development of treatment alternatives in the community.

Admission and discharge procedures, commitment laws, the lack of privacy and the loss of dignity in many psychiatric hospitals as a result of overcrowding of facilities and lack of funds, and the little or lack of involvement in community mental health need to be addressed in Latin America. The time has come for an examination of what is happening in psychiatric hospitals and to patients in those hospitals, and for the institution of change. The time has also come for mental health professionals to turn their attention to the mental health needs of their communities. Only a few projects have been reported that deal with community treatment and psychiatric rehabilitation programs (Busnello et al. 1975; Climent and Arango 1980; Eisenberg 1980; Fernandez Bruno and Gabay 1997; González Uzcátegui and Levav 1991; Organización Mundial de la Salud 1984). One interesting project, organized by PAHO in cooperation with the Calgary World Health Organization Center for Research and Training in Mental Health, has involved training police officers in the management of mentally ill patients in the community. This program has been quite successful in several countries in the English-speaking Caribbean (Arboleda-Flórez et al. 1997), and materials have been translated into Spanish. Finally, the time has come for psychiatrists and other mental health professionals to become activists to address the sociopolitical foundations of violence and other ills in their societies (Rouillon 1997). In this regard, national associations of mental health professionals, for example, could ask for official status as nongovernmental organizations. This is a new development in Colombia and elsewhere in Latin America, where nongovernmental organizations have lately been requesting that the general public be represented in discussions of major national, political, and social issues (Useche De Brill 1998).

Ethical Considerations

As previously mentioned, the ethical discourse in Latin America departs from the Judeo-Christian (mostly Catholic) approach brought by settlers from Spain and Portugal (Lavados et al. 1990; Mainetti 1989). In a leading treatise on ethics, for example, ethics is defined as "the study of the goodness and evil in human conduct" (Varga 1990, p. 5) (our translation). In Catholic ethics, morality is the foundation of our actions. More recently, however, a humanistic ethical discourse has entered the field of ethics in Latin America, mostly through translations of North American or European books (Scorer and Wing 1983). This is inevitable as ethicists begin to grapple with issues of abortion, euthanasia, organ donation, reproductive technology, and allocation of resources and with the ethics of physicians in health systems that impinge on the physician-patient relationship and confidentiality (Drane 1993). Normative ethics, according to some authors, may not have the answers to the dilemmas of modern medicine. These authors advocate a case-by-case approach, situationally based, in which rights and duties are explored within a covenant joining the parties (Veatch 1981).

Intense work is taking place in the area of bioethics in countries such as Colombia, Mexico, Argentina, and Chile. In relation to psychiatry and mental health ethics, ethical discourse follows lines not too different from those followed in North America or Europe. Figueroa (1994), for example, argued that psychiatry is limited to unmasking falsifications of self-recognition in the moral life of the patient. He proposed that the issue in psychiatric ethics is access to true discourse and that the true ethical value in psychiatry is veracity. Some other authors have reflected on the softness of psychiatric diagnoses, the side effects of psychiatric drugs, and the legitimacy of psychotherapy as it invades the privacy of the patient (Dorr Zegers 1993). Others have pondered on the relationship between economic factors and ethical dictates as well as the crosscurrents between ethics and psychology in relation to motivation, character structures, the nature of the moral act, and moral responsibility and culpability (Valenzuela 1992).

On the other hand, a dialectic has also been developed in psychiatric ethics whereby protection of the patient's liberty and rights is considered fundamental to the physician-patient relationship and to the routines of daily psychiatric work (Cassiers 1988). An ethics of rights, as defended by Brody (1993), has in fact permeated the psychiatric ethical discourse in Latin America (Taborda 1996). Several authors have explored this theme and asked whether psychiatry can truly answer ethical questions of liberty and rights when double allegiances seem inevitable and even obligatory by law (Lewis 1991).

An ethics of rights at the very basic level of human decency, however, is evident in the Declaration of Caracas (González Uzcátegui and Levav 1991), which states:

> The resources, care and treatment provided must: safeguard, in a definite form, the personal dignity and the civil and human rights [of the patients]; be based on rational criteria and be technically appropriate; [and] aim at keeping the patient in the community of origin.

In another section, the declaration calls for legislative change:

> 4. That mental health legislation in each country be modified so that it: ensures the respect of civil and human rights of mental patients, and promotes the organization of community mental health services where rights are also protected.

González Uzcátegui and Levav (1991) wrote that on many occasions, mentally ill patients have their rights abrogated or abused by virtue of their conditions and that this is more obvious among chronically ill patients in psychiatric hospitals, to which many are committed without medical reason. In many other instances their rights are openly violated without clear recognition by the perpetrators of their wrongdoing. González Uzcátegui and Levav (1991) concluded that for these reasons "it could be stated that the law does not protect the rights of patients with mental illness so there is a need to spell them out and clearly state how the law should protect them" (p. 105) (our translation).

Conclusions

In this chapter, we reviewed cultural and ethical issues and the system for the delivery of psychiatric services in Latin America. Emphasis was placed on specific areas that we believe are salient to an understanding of the lives of Latin Americans, their cultural values, their problems, and their ethical discourse as it pertains to psychiatric problems and the delivery of psychiatric services in the region. We hope that clustering this many issues has not led to oversimplification and the loss of recognition of their uniqueness in the different countries of Latin America.

References

Arboleda-Flórez J, Copithorne M: Mental Health Law and Practice. Toronto, Carswell, 1994

Arboleda-Flórez J, Crisanti A, Holley H: The Police Officer as a Primary Mental Health Officer. Washington, DC, Pan American Health Organization, 1997

Basaglia F: L'Instituzione negata. Turin, Italy, Einaudi, 1968

Bongaarts J: Demographic consequences of declining fertility. Science 282:419–420, 1998

Brody EB: Biomedical Technology and Human Rights. Dartmouth, England, UNESCO Publishing, 1993

Busnello E, Lewin I, Ruschel S, et al: Projeto de um sistema comunitario de saude. Pôrto Alegre, Brazil, Centro Médico Social São José de Murialdo; Secretaria de Saude de Rio Grande do Sul, 1975

Canino IA, Canino GJ: Psychiatric care of Puerto Ricans, in Culture, Ethnicity and Mental Illness. Edited by Gaw EC. Washington, DC, American Psychiatric Press, 1993, pp 467–499

Cassiers L: Questions éthiques en psychiatrie. Louvain Médecine 107:519–527, 1988

Climent CE, Arango MV: Estrategias para la extensión de los servicios de salud mental en los paises en desarrollo, I: descripción del proyecto. Acta Psiquiátrica y Psicológica de América Latina 26:48–53, 1980

De La Cancela V, Guarnaccia PJ, Carillo E: Psychosocial distress among Latinos: a critical analysis of *ataques de nervios*. Humanity and Society 10:431–447, 1986

División de Salud Mental del Ministerio de Sanidad y Asistencia Social de Venezuela: Anteproyecto de ley de protección y atención integral a las personas con trastornos mentales. Caracas, División de Salud Mental del Ministerio de Sanidad y Asistencia Social de Venezuela, 1993

Dorr Zegers O: El desafío ético en la psiquiatría. Rev Med Chil 121:811–818, 1993

Drane JF: Como ser un buen médico. Bogotá, San Pablo, 1993

Eisenberg C: Mental health in Honduras: the community approach. World Forum 1:72–77, 1980

Fernandez Bruno MD, Gabay PM: Rehabilitación y resocialización de enfermos mentales en una casa de medio camino. Poster presented at the 4th International Congress of Psychiatry, Buenos Aires, Argentina, May 1997

Figueroa G: Los fundamentos de la bioética desde la ética psiquiátrica. Revista Chilena Neuro-Psiquiátrica 32:19–26, 1994

Fox E (ed): Media and Politics in Latin America: The Struggle for Democracy. London, Sage, 1988

González Uzcátegui R, Levav I: Reestructuración de la atención psiquiátrica: bases conceptuales y guías para su implementación. Washington, DC, Organización Panamericana de la Salud, 1991

Guerrero R: Epidemiology of violence in the Americas: the case of Colombia, in Poverty & Inequality: Annual World Bank Conference on Development in Latin America and the Caribbean: 1996. Edited by Burki SJ, Aiyer S-R, Hommes R. Washington DC, World Bank, 1998, pp 95–100

Helman CG: Culture, Health and Illness. Oxford, Butterworth-Heinemann, 1994

Hippocrates: Airs, waters, places, in The Challenge of Epidemiology. Edited by Buck C, Llopis A, Najera E, et al. Washington, DC, Pan American Health Organization, 1988, pp 18–19

Hollingsworth EJ: Mental health services in England: the 1990s. Int J Law Psychiatry 19:309–325, 1996

Homicidios no Sao Paolo. Folha de São Paulo, March 31, 1998, p 1

Hufford DJ, Chilton M: Politics, spirituality, and environmental healing, in The Ecology of Health. Edited by Chesworth J. Thousand Oaks, CA, Sage, 1996, pp 59–71

Kiev A: Transcultural Psychiatry. Harmondsworth, England, Penguin, 1972

Lavados M, Monge JI, Quintana C, et al. (eds): Problemas contemporaneos en bioética. Santiago de Chile, Chile, Ediciónes Universidad Católica de Chile, 1990

Lewis A: Dilemmas in psychiatry. Psychol Med 21:581–585, 1991

Lolas F: Ecología psiquiátrica, in Psiquiatría. Edited by Vidal G, Alarcon RD. Buenos Aires, Editorial Médica Panamericana, 1986, pp 97–98

Mainetti JA: Ética médica: introducción histórica. La Plata, Argentina, Quiron, 1989

Merrill FE: Society and Culture. Englewood Cliffs, NJ, Prentice-Hall, 1961

Mezzich JE, Lewis-Fernandez R: Cultural considerations in psychopathology, in Psychiatry, Vol 1. Edited by Tasman A, Kay J, Lieberman JA. Philadelphia, PA, WB Saunders, 1997, pp 563–571

Minayo MC: A violência social sob a perspectiva da saúde pública, in O impacto da violência social sobre a saúde. Escola Nacional de Saúde Pública, Cadernos de Saúude Pública 10 (suppl 1):7–18, 1994

Opler MK, Rennie TAC: Culture, Psychiatry and Human Values. Springfield, IL, Charles C Thomas, 1956

Organización Mundial de la Salud: Atención de salud mental en los paises en desarrollo: análisis críticos de los resultados de las investigaciónes. Informe de un grupo de estudio de la OMS (Serie de informes técnicos No. 698). Geneva, Organización Mundial de la Salud, 1984

Organización Panamericana de la Salud: Salud mental en el nivel primario de atención: estudio de una muestra de pacientes en seis paises centroamericanos. Washington, DC, Organización Panamericana de la Salud, 1995

Pan American Health Organization: Health Conditions in the Americas, Vol 1 (Scientific Publication No 524). Washington, DC, Pan American Health Organization, 1990, pp 207–212

Pan American Health Organization: Declaration of the Inter-American Conference on Society, Violence and Health. Washington, DC, Pan American Health Organization, 1994

Province of Ontario: Mental Health Act, R.S.O. 1990, c. M.7, in Ontario Consent and Capacity Legislation. Aurora, ON, Canada, Canada Law Books, 1990, pp 1–36

Ridgway P: From asylums to communities: a historical perspective on changing environments of care, in Psychiatry, Vol 2. Edited by Tasman A, Kay J, Lieberman JA. Philadelphia, PA, WB Saunders, 1997, pp 1751–1769

Rouillon F: L'Épidémiologie des troubles agressifs, in Criminologie et psychiatrie. Edited by Albernhe T. Paris, Ellipses, 1997, pp 450–454

Rubel AJ: The epidemiology of a folk illness: *susto* in Hispanic America, in Culture, Disease, and Healing: Studies in Medical Anthropology. Edited by Landy D. New York, Macmillan, 1977, pp 119–128

Scorer G, Wing A: Problemas éticos en medicina. Barcelona, Doyma, 1983

Seguin CA: La esperanza y la fe, in Psiquiatría. Edited by Vidal G, Alarcon RD. Buenos Aires, Editorial Médica Panamericana, 1986, pp 129–130

Spooner B: The evil eye in the Middle East, in Witchcraft: Confessions and Accusations. Edited by Douglass M. London, Tavistock, 1970, pp 311–319

Swanson GE: On explanations of social interaction. Sociometry 28:101–123, 1965

Taborda JGV: Psiquiatria legal, in Rotinas em psiquiatria. Edited by Taborda JGV, Prado-Lima P, D'Arrigo Busnello E. Pôrto Alegre, Brazil, Artes Médicas, 1996, pp 280–296

Underwood P, Underwood Z: New spells for old: expectations and realities of Western medicine in a remote tribal society in Yemen, Arabia, in Changing Disease Patterns and Human Behaviour. Edited by Stanley NF, Joshe RA. London, Academic Press, 1981, pp 271–297

Useche De Brill I: Innovations in the rendering of services by the Colombian Confederation of Nongovernmental Organizations, in Poverty and Inequality: Annual World Bank Conference on Development in Latin America and the Caribbean: 1996. Edited by Burki SJ, Aiyer S-R, Hommes R. Washington, DC, World Bank, 1998, pp 301–305

Valenzuela GE: Ética: introducción a su problemática y su historia. Mexico City, McGraw-Hill/Interamericana de México, 1992

Varga AC: Bioética: problemas principales. Bogotá, Paulinas, 1990

Veatch RM: A Theory of Medical Ethics. New York, Basic Books, 1981

Zeman PM, Schwartz HI: Hospitalization: voluntary and involuntary, in Principles and Practice of Forensic Psychiatry. Edited by Rosner R. New York, Chapman & Hall, 1994, pp 111–118

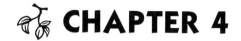 CHAPTER 4

A West Mediterranean Perspective

Prof. Juan J. López-Ibor, Jr.
Dr. M. Dolores Crespo

The goals of ethics are universal. Therefore, individual, cultural, or social differences should not be excuses, as they are often considered, for unacceptable behavior. In fact, this universal aspect of ethics is stressed in the Declaration of Madrid of the World Psychiatric Association (see the Appendix to this book), which states: "Although there may be cultural, social, and national differences, the need for ethical conduct and continual review of ethical standards is universal." As a consequence, the study of ethics in a specific historical and cultural context, such as Mediterranean Europe, must be considered a way to contribute to the development of a universal ethic.

Psychiatric ethics are not different from ethics in general. Professionals, being members of a specific society, adopt ethical principles in accordance with the society to which they belong. Braceland (1969) put forward the notion that doctors, as citizens, must be ethical and act according to the established and accepted standards applied to all citizens. Clouser (1973) considered medical ethics to be ethics applied to a particular aspect of life, namely medicine.

Cultures are defined by their values and peculiarities—among them, ethics. Those ethics are assumed to belong to individual cultures and are part of the identity of every social group. However, social diversity, multicultural-ism, and the concern about ethical and social diversity in modern society make it even more necessary to adopt universal and common ethical values. Delving into the diversity of different cultures and ethics is essential to harmonize equality with difference, homogeneity with diversity, and individual beliefs with social norms—that is, to find ethical values that are universal for all persons and social groups.

The Individual and Society

Traditional Mediterranean Ethos

Ethos is the way in which individuals, cultural groups, and nations' peoples interpret their own history, their social world, and their physical environment to formulate opinions and convictions, which are the background for ethical behavior. Every culture is the manifestation of a specific way of life.

According to Gracia and Jonsen (1998), there are two main types of ethics: one based on the notions of goodness or virtue (Aristotelian ethics) and one based on principles (Anglo-Saxon [i.e., referring to English-speaking peoples] ethics). In Anglo-Saxon ethics, priority is given to the rights of the individual, particularly freedom, with only one limitation, which is that harm must not be caused to third parties.

Mediterranean culture is made up of ethical traditions of diverse origins. The oldest tradition is Greek, of which Aristotelian philosophy is the most representative (Aristotle 1990). Aristotelian ethics were adopted by Rome and contributed to the development of Roman law.

Combined in Mediterranean ethics are the Asian idea of duty toward the community and the concept in Asian and Arab cultures of protection of a person's dignity. Mediterranean ethics are centered more on social aspects, and the individual is seen as inserted in a social group. Mediterranean ethics, like all ethical traditions, are based on the idea of goodness and respect toward men and women; more specifically, they are centered on the concepts of virtue and vice. In Mediterranean ethics, freedom and duty are put at the same level.

The Mediterranean ethos was well described by the Spanish philosopher Unamuno y Jugo in his work *El sentimiento trágico de la vida* ("The tragic feeling of life"). This ethos is based on the struggle of the forces of nature, of society, and of the character of individuals, a concept at odds with the American feeling of a happy ending (A. Jonsen, "American Ethos and American Bioethics," Madrid, Spain, 1998).

People of the Mediterranean have a great sensitivity for virtues such as trust and friendship, which characterize particular relationships, including the doctor-patient relationship. Accordingly, the patient wants and seeks a doctor to be trusted in, more than a doctor who guides himself or herself by duties and rights to fulfil preestablished norms, as is the case in Anglo-Saxon cultures.

European Ethos

López Ibor Sr. (1965) called attention to the difficulties of defining *Europe* in a precise way. It is a part of the world full of variety and dispersion, with geographic and historical limits that are not well defined and that have led to many discussions among intellectuals.

In spite of this, it is relatively easy to define *European*, used to describe the lifestyle of individuals in Europe and the society to which they belong. The concept of European is the result of many cultures. To be European is to adopt the historic attitude that led to the birth of Europe, an attitude characterized by the search for new ways of life.

In Europe, there has always been a strong impulse to integrate other forms and experiences of life. The ability to assimilate, together with a spirit to progress, to take risks in search of perfection, has shaped the ethos of Europe.

Technology was born in Europe. It is the consequence of the human ability to imitate and check what takes place in nature once religious fear or admiration, leading to the seeing in every natural event participation of a divinity, has been overcome. Technology is developed to solve everyday problems and to advance world unification. Although technology permits the meeting of common needs, technology without humanitarian concern produces dissatisfaction. Modern Europeans need to cultivate the essences of their nature and their values if they are not to be estranged by technology.

Modern Mediterranean Ethics

In the Mediterranean, ethics is considered a rational science, in which common ethical contents rather than moral differences are identified. In the Anglo-Saxon world, by contrast, ethics is not a rational science but involves consensus and social contracts. In this form of ethics, coming to agreement in the face of different opinions becomes essential, and laws are used as a last resort to resolve conflicts. In Mediterranean ethics, on the other hand, there is less tendency to debate or jointly deliberate to reach agreement, with the result that there is less concern about problems of minorities.

In Mediterranean ethics, a distance is kept from religious, political, and secular fundamentalism. Avoided are identification between religion and state (there is separation of church and state), politics as religion (there exist a multiparty system, political pluralism, and free and rational public-opinion debates), and extreme liberalism that excludes ethics from public life (politics must be guided by a rational ethics).

Rather than being politically affiliated, Mediterranean ethics involve political ideals, which should be respected by all social powers: respect for private property and promotion of fair distribution of wealth. This form of ethics is therefore neither conservative nor progressive. Mediterranean ethics are historically prescriptive and not descriptive; as in bioethics today, perspectives from all periods and cultures are incorporated.

> Mediterranean ethics goes beyond personalism and although it is radical and social, it insists on the collective character, on the group, on the need for communication and dialogue, on cultural identity, on the duties each one has toward the community, on the need for social justice and worldwide distribution as an essential element of the virtue of justice . . . of course parting from a sine qua non condition of the dignity of each human being. (Elósegui 1998) (our translation)

Modern medical terms reflect this duality. In Anglo-Saxon cultures, there are doctors called *primary care physicians*, implying the notion of types of care (primary versus specialty care). In Mediterranean cultures, the same physicians are called *family doctors* or *community doctors*, implying a role of taking care of a social structure (the family or the community).

Medical Ethics

Ethics of Welfare

Traditional medical ethics, stemming from Hippocratic writings, is an ethics of welfare. The goals and duties of doctors are expressed as much in terms of the well-being of their patients as of the harm to be avoided.

However, the way of understanding nature among classical Greeks forced Hippocratic doctors to deny medical care to incurable patients. To care for a patient without being able to restore the patient to health and restore his or her well-being is a confrontation with nature *(physis)*, and this was considered immoral (Vintró 1972). Today, in a more or less conspicuous way, many practitioners adopt a similar attitude toward patients with certain terminal illnesses or incurable patients such as mentally retarded persons (Barcia 1992).

Contributions of Christianity

The ethical model of welfare was enriched by the Alexandrian notion of philanthropy, based on the following principle: *where there is love to art (of healing), there is also love to mankind.* With the addition of Christianity, this medical moral concept included the spiritual life. Therefore, Christian practitioners were obliged to deal also with the spiritual lives of their patients. In this way, the principle of welfare was born and the obligation of giving medical care to incurable patients was adopted, resulting in unselfish treatment and regular medical care, essentially driven by charity (Beauchamp and McCullough 1987).

The basic principles of welfare ethics still hold and are present in recent deontological medical codes because doctors resist giving up their traditional roles as benefactors (Gafo 1986). In this context, the doctor is perceived and behaves as a good father, in whom the patient must trust, convinced that the doctor will act adequately for his or her benefit. For this, the doctor must increase to the maximum his or her own medical knowledge, assume a series of obligations, and undertake promotion of virtues. In a similar way, the patient is seen as a minor who must bestow trust on the practitioner, in the security that the actions of the practitioner will be the right ones. The tie that binds both is friendship, medically understood (Barcia 1979; Lain Entralgo 1984).

American influence, with its strong emphasis on autonomy and individualism, led to the ethics of autonomy. In 1973, the American Hospital Association adopted the Patient's Bill of Rights, drafted by the American Association for Consumers. This bill of rights was later accepted by the rest of the Western countries, Spain among them, introducing the ethics of autonomy (Gaylin 1978).

In the ethics of autonomy, the patient is considered an autonomous human being, adult and free and consequently able to make his or her own decisions. The values and beliefs of the patient are the background for the moral responsibilities of the doctor. When the patient's values collide with those of the doctor, the fundamental responsibility of the doctor is to respect and facilitate the patient's self-determination in the making of decisions regarding his or her destiny in relation to medicine.

As a consequence, doctors must truly inform patients about all possible diagnoses and treatments so that patients are able to come to decisions. The basic element of this new way of establishing the doctor-patient relationship is informed consent (López-Ibor Jr. and Crespo Hervás 1996). Autonomy is linked to the liberty to choose and the ability to assume responsibility for one's own acts—in other words, liberty from pressures of any kind and the ability to rule one's own life (Gracia 1986, 1991).

From this perspective, the doctor-patient relationship is defined in new terms, some of them not easy. With regard to confidentiality, for example, the main problem is knowing whether confidentiality is an absolute or a relative obligation. Most authors are inclined to consider confidentiality a relative duty, among other reasons because it must not be maintained when the illness may affect the well-being of third parties. Barcia and Crespo in Spain (1998) state that confidentiality should always be absolute and should therefore never be violated.

Ethics of Equity

The way psychiatric care is delivered and the way psychiatrists relate to patients are changing very quickly. Economic factors in medicine have accelerated these changes. The need for equal access to health care resources for all patients, including those with mental illness, and the principle of equity in a period of intrinsic and extrinsic cost limitations in health care are leading to a third stage of bioethics, which has been called *ethics of management* but should be called *ethics of equity*.

Integration of psychiatric care. Psychiatrists have been fighting for years for the integration of psychiatric care into general health care and for recognition of the role of general health care professionals in detecting and managing psychiatric disturbances in general medical practice and psychosocial aspects of nonpsychiatric diseases. Part of this effort is the training of other doctors and health care professionals for these tasks. As a consequence, psychiatrists are now connected with new medical and social structures. Because of the competition for resources (e.g., beds, professionals, space in community centers, research funding), psychiatrists have had to learn to use more medical language and less psychiatric terminology to permit the growth of the specialty. With the introduction of neuroleptics and the closing of psychiatric hospitals, mental illness has become visible on every street downtown in big cities all over the world and is often associated with alcohol and drug abuse. Resisting the pressure to consider this aspect a social rather than a medical issue, while maintaining access to social services for psychiatric patients, is also important.

The Spanish mental health care system has evolved during the last 20 years around the following points:

♦ Full integration of psychiatric care into general health care, acknowledged in the General Law of Health. In the past, psychiatric care was provided through welfare, outside the social security system. A slow evolution led finally to full integration in a national health system model. Only hypnosis and psychoanalysis are excluded from the care provided for mentally ill patients.

♦ Removal of particular consideration of the legal situation of patients with mental illness. In the past, a very detailed and efficient law regulated the admission and discharge of mentally ill patients. This has been replaced by a single item in the Civil Code. This change initially raised concerns among psychiatrists, but now it should be seen as an effective way of integrating the care of mentally ill patients with that of other patients, as well as a way of avoiding the stigma of mental illness.

♦ Decentralization of health care administration. Different systems and levels of care have been put into practice in different regions. In general, there has been an effort to create community mental health centers and to close old institutions.

Economic aspects of health care. The end of the Second World War paved the way for a revolution in the practice of medicine. This fact was not recognized until economic factors led to a conflict between what is theoretically possible and what can be achieved in reality. Economic factors disrupt the intimate and traditional doctor-patient relationship.

The past period of economic prosperity allowed essential developments in medicine in Europe and in other parts of the world. Medical care has become accessible to every citizen in many countries; in the past, only individuals who could afford care obtained it. New and expensive technologies have been developed and large institutions such as modern hospitals have been established. New professions have been incorporated into medicine and there has been development of teamwork. Biomedical research has been financed and has led to important findings. Finally, resources have been allocated for the training of physicians and specialists, training that is longer and more complicated than in the past.

With the increase in health care costs came the negative impact of economic aspects on the doctor-patient relationship. Doctor strikes took place, for the first time, in Italy in the late 1960s, and since then have occurred in many other countries.

The increase in or imbalance of costs is partially due to developments in modern medicine. Health care itself is increasingly expensive. Further, because acute diseases are better controlled, there are more chronically ill patients requiring care. The demand for health care has increased because of the aging of populations. Finally, in social security systems, the change in the population pyramid means that the population paying for health care is smaller than the population incurring the expenses.

In most of Europe, health care is state administered or state controlled. For instance, Spain has a social security system, which covers almost 100% of the population and includes free medical care, in the form of a national health system. The system evolved from a system financed by employers and employees to one in which an increased proportion of the budget was covered by taxes.

Resources to be invested in health care are limited. The first one to ask for limits was Jimmy Carter, during his first public speech, in 1977, after assuming the United States presidency. Carter called for a ceiling of 7% of the gross national product. He claimed that too much spending in this area would decrease investments in education and care of the environment, which would lead to deterioration of health.

The fact that more is not better is evident when health indices are compared. Life expectancy is lower in the United States (around 69 years for men and 72 years for women), where more than 14% of the gross national product is dedicated to health care and where medical treatment is of the best in the world, than in Japan, France, Italy, or Spain (around 72–73 years for men and 79–80 years for women), which spends less. Diet is considered an important factor, but the so-called Mediterranean diet is very different from the Japanese one. Recently, importance has been given to the structure of the family and the way in which children are raised. Therefore, many factors play a role in health, and not only in health care, and resources are needed to investigate and promote them.

Access to full health care for every individual is no longer possible. In the United States, which takes the capitalistic approach, there were almost 40.9 million people without insurance in 1995 (*Business Review*, March 27, 1995). This number grew from 34.4 million in 1991, in spite of Medicare and Medicaid. In other countries that take the European approach, equivalent numbers of people are on waiting lists. These two approaches are spontaneous but highly unfair ways of controlling costs.

Callahan (1991) called for limits on health care, just as there are limits, accepted by doctors, to what should be done for individual patients with terminal illness. Kilner (1992) analyzed the ethical principles usually applied when making decisions about when to treat and when not to treat. The conclusion was that all principles are ethically unacceptable. Most of them would even violate the constitutions of most modern democratic societies that protect minority groups. For instance, no ethical principle supports the denial of liver transplantation for a chronic alcoholic individual whose condition has deteriorated. Kilner's solution is most uncomfortable: When resources (in this case, livers for transplanting) are few, a lottery should be used to determine who receives them.

Management techniques are being introduced in Europe in a more acceptable way than in the United States. The goal of cost control is not considered in isolation from other goals—specifically, quality assurance and equity. Management has three other components.

The first additional component is information—what physicians do, how patients behave, and, more important, long-term outcomes of medical interventions. Quality-of-life studies also play a role in this part of management.

The second additional component is consensus. Doctors could probably reach a consensus on diagnosis. The *Diagnostic and Statistical Manual of Mental Disorders*, 4th Edition (DSM-IV) (American Psychiatric Association 1994) and the *International Statistical Classification of Diseases and Related Health Problems*, 10th Revision (ICD-10) (World Health Organization 1992) are evidence of how we psychiatrists can have a common language, common treatments, and common measures of outcome. It is only we who can say when a patient should be admitted, or when he or she should receive a particular expensive drug rather than an inexpensive one, or when he or she should undergo an expensive brain-imaging examination. Health care economists, the administration, or health maintenance organizations or insurance companies will then have to calculate the economic impact and make appropriate decisions. Information will help physicians, economists, and policy makers to reach a consensus on what is more appropriate for the individual and for the social group as a whole.

The third additional component of management is a new medical ethics, in which the consequences of the individualistic and paternalistic traditional "compassionate" doctor-patient relationship are overcome. The social contract on health and disease issues that was introduced at the end of the Second World War worked, or seemed to work, for a couple of decades. Now the discussion is louder and broader, and it will lead to a more stable social contract, but only if the voices of physicians are heard.

New Challenges to the Doctor-Patient Relationship

Radical changes have occurred in the doctor-patient relationship in recent years, leading to new ethical demands by professionals. On the one hand, these changes are a consequence of the triumph of the ideas of the French

Revolution and of the secularization and democratization of modern societies. On the other hand, these changes have been determined by economic forces, which at the same time have allowed the extraordinary progress of medicine in the last decades and the universalization of medical care, introducing a third party in the doctor-patient relationship (López-Ibor Jr. 1997). This third party is health economy, and it is precisely what makes it possible for patients to go to a doctor in the form of national health services or private insurance companies.

On the other hand, health has become a consumer good, and the doctor-patient relationship is established in contractual terms. This means that patients await benefits for which they are paying, and if they are not satisfied with the results, they can legally act against their doctors. It is the patient who determines medical activities. Many of the current requests, such as for sterilization, nontherapeutic abortion, or "cosmetic psychopharmacology" (Kramer 1993), have nothing to do with medicine as an activity directed toward the healing of illness. Closely related to this is the so-called patient-physician covenant (Crawshaw et al. 1995), more and more used in the defense of clinical activity in the face of political, economic, or judicial pressure or pressures within the medical profession (e.g., those arising from excessive greed) (Crawshaw 1996).

The Problem of Truth in Psychiatry

The problem of truth in research and psychiatric practice should be resolved in the personal relationship. For a long time, psychiatrists felt uncomfortable with the problem of truth, although it was enclosed in the definition of the delusional idea. This is why the classical definition was replaced by the definition of the delusional idea based on structure, not on content as in the case of German psychiatry (Gruhle 1929; Jaspers 1955; Schneider 1963). In a certain sense, from this perspective, the fidelity of a spouse is irrelevant in the definition of the delusional idea of jealousy.

Reintroduction and analysis of the problem of truth are the way to overcome the crisis of psychopathology. Truth is not a unanimous concept. There is logical truth, which is the opposite of falseness, and metaphysical truth, the opposite of the illusory, the unreal (Ferrater Mora 1979). Since Aristotle, truth has been considered the adaptation of the intellect to the thing. However, Heidegger (1953) analyzed the concept of truth in the writings of pre-Socratic philosophers and established truth as a process of discovery, of revealing the hidden that opens up to us (the truth as *aletheia*). This concept of truth is similar to the process of psychotherapeutic research—the process of revealing the hidden meaning of neurotic symptoms. There is still more: according to Heidegger, truth comes together in freedom. The essence of truth is freedom—freedom to leave as they are, whatever they are, the things and people as they reveal themselves. Truth has therefore an interpersonal character; it is an interpersonal process (Heidegger 1953).

Kunz (1954–1955), trying to increase the knowledge of delusional ideas, looked for ideas held by healthy individuals that were similar to delusional ideas of persons with schizophrenia and found only one—the idea of death, in which operate the same defense mechanisms. This is the opposite of a healthy, constructive, realistic attitude, an attitude of humbleness and tolerance.

One of the basic characteristics of the delusional patient is the inability to tolerate ambiguity. This characteristic enslaves the patient to an unavoidable certainty. A patient said that if he did not accept his delusions, he would have to deal with an unbearable anguish, because he could not believe nor accept the rest of his experiences. Ambiguity derives from the fact that the human being lives in two worlds, the common world *(koinos cosmos)* and the world of his or her fantasies and dreams *(idios cosmos)* (Kuhn 1963). It is the same ambiguity that exists in the body (described by Merleau-Ponty [1945]), the ambiguity of being able to simultaneously say "I am" and "I have" (Marcel 1955). Ambiguity is a radical of human existence and therefore of knowledge. The intolerance of delusional patients leads them to alienate an important part of their psychic lives that no longer belongs to them but belongs to others—to the ones who shout, rummage, or send rays to injure their bodies or invade their thoughts.

Blankenburg (1965) made an interpretation of the delusional patient from a similar perspective. To try to clarify how delusional patients' ideas differ from those of nondelusional individuals, he had his patients write poems. Blankenburg (1965) presented a beautiful poem by one of his patients that contained metaphors and images extraordinarily similar to those in a poem by Rilke. Blankenburg wrote that the difference between nondelusional and delusional individuals lies not in the content of their poetry but in the writers themselves. Once the (nondelusional) poet has finished his or her work, the poet hurries to the editor for publication, whereas the delusional patient throws the work away or abandons it and does not even keep it for himself or herself. Paranoia is to be found not in the content but in the individual (Hillman 1985).

From this perspective, the falseness of the delusional idea becomes clearer: It is both a "false truth," a wolf in sheep's clothing, which imposes itself as a certainty, and an autistic truth, inaccessible in the present ambiguity. The problem is not whether the idea of jealousy is certain but rather the lack of mutual confidence, which hinders the jealous person from going beyond his or her own jealousy. It cannot be overlooked that these thoughts have a very important practical outcome. For example, McNaughton's Rules on insanity defense, which have prevailed for decades in Anglo-Saxon countries, are based on the rigid application of a wrongly interpreted concept of truth. If a delusional, jealous man kills his wife or her presumed or real lover, he must pay the penalty because whether the infidelity was real or not, the crime is not justified and the patient, like any other citizen, knows this. McNaughton, a man with schizophrenia who spent almost all of his life in London's Bethlem Hospital, would have been executed if the rules that bear his name had been applied to him.

Heidegger's approach (Heidegger 1953) has important implications for psychiatry. It is clear that the process of the truth corresponds with the psychotherapeutic process, in which the interpersonal relationship is the basis for knowledge.

It has, on the other hand, strong ties to ethical and religious traditions. The religious root of Freudian thought has not been unperceived. López-Ibor Jr. (1975) referred to the gnostic perspective. The implicit Manichaeanism in gnostic dualism provides a solid ethical basis because it allows the existence of two natures, one of which justifies evil and can be, must be, finally gained by the other one, although in the course of a war some battles may be lost. The problem of evil, the structure of evil, has been considered the basic problem of science, at least the social sciences (Becker 1980), because science is in itself gnostic. But the Freudian thinking is gnostic not only because it is scientific but also because it embraces a mystic Jewish tradition (Bakan 1964). The reading of sacred Jewish texts depends on an interpretation, which is a re-creation. Hebrew, like other Semitic languages, has no written vowels, and vowels must be inserted during the reading of a text if the text is to be understood. The attempt must be made in this process to remain true to the original text and to the sense of the text as a whole. Reading is therefore an exercise in revealing the word.

The French philosopher Marlène Zarader (1990) was highly critical of Heidegger's philosophy, with his unacknowledged debt to the biblical tradition. The fact that the man who delved into the roots of modern thinking in classical Greece, at the time and in the place of the Logos, of oral thought, could neither think nor say the essential element of his speech is surprising. Zarader's thesis was that Heidegger's philosophy has a strong Hebraic influence. The texts go far beyond analogy. Heidegger was as much a poet as was a prophet in the Bible, and Heidegger's poetry is an interpretation in the sense of re-creation of the text.

In scientific research, in the process of obtaining knowledge, there is always a personal element that must be displayed in a context. In a speech at Complutense University in Madrid, Karl Popper described the three ethical principles of the search for truth based on rational dialogue (K. Popper, "Una nueva ética profesional," 1992 [the following is our translation]):

1. *The principle of reliability:* Maybe I am wrong and maybe you are right, but we may, of course, both be wrong.

2. *The principle of rational dialogue:* We want to critically . . . proof our reasons against and for our varied theories. This critical attitude to which we are obliged to adhere is part of our intellectual responsibility.

3. *The principle of approach to the truth with the aid of debate:* We can almost always approach truth with the aid of impersonal (and objective) critical discussions, and this way we can almost always improve our understanding, even in those cases in which we do not reach an agreement.

It is extraordinary that these three principles are epistemological and at the same time they are also ethical principles. They imply, among other things, tolerance: if I can learn something from you and if I want to learn, for the sake of searching for the truth, not only do I have to tolerate you as a person, but I have to potentially recognize you as an equal; the potential unity of humanity and the potential equality of all human beings is a prerequirement to our will to rationally carry out a dialogue. The principle according to which we can learn a lot from discussion is of even greater importance, even when we do not reach an agreement. A rational dialogue can help us throw light on errors, even our own errors.

When applying all this to the doctor-patient relationship and to such a relationship in extreme cases—the relationship between a psychiatrist and a patient with mental illness—and as stated in the Declaration of Madrid, one must conclude that there is only one model for authentic relationships between human beings and that this model must be applied to all situations. In other words, the relationship between a doctor and a patient does not differ from the relationship between a teacher and his or her students, nor from the relationships in a group of researchers, nor in fact from relationships among human beings in general. All are based on tolerance and on giving the other all possible opportunities.

The problem of truth in medicine refers to the real doctor-patient relationship, to the revealing of the significance of symptoms, to the research into negative and self-destructive habits, to the revealing of the sense of an existence, to the foundations of mutual confidence, and to the desire and effort to improve—improvement that in the most favorable cases involves achieving a higher level of authenticity and greater liberty.

New Criteria for Informed Consent

For many years in Spain and other Mediterranean European countries, the majority of physicians made decisions on behalf of their patients, considering that this was always for their patients' well-being. This form of paternalism was in keeping with the social and family structures prevalent in those years. Because this paternalistic conception of the doctor-patient relationship is deeply rooted in European culture, above all in the Mediterranean, several authors wrote that it would be unwise to introduce abrupt changes.

Nevertheless, social changes—especially in Spain since the late 1970s, coinciding with and as a consequence of the country's democratization—affected the doctor-patient relationship. The change to a relationship in which the patient has more autonomy has been abrupt and often precipitate. Furthermore, in Spain the purpose of this change was not very well articulated, and the change was to some degree forced.

Informed consent must be understood as a gradual process that is carried out in the core of the doctor-patient relationship. Through informed consent, the patient receives from the doctor enough information to participate actively in decision making regarding his or her treatment. Imparting information in a caregiving relationship is a duty of the professional and is as important as any other of his or her duties.

Informed consent should be applicable to psychiatric practice in the same way that it is applicable in everyday practice, although the conditions of patients with mental disorders can make application especially difficult.

The information given to the psychiatric patient regarding his or her diagnosis and treatment and the request for consent together permit systematic evaluation of the patient's competency. Not all mentally ill patients are incompetent, and those who are incompetent are rarely so during the entire course of their illness. Therefore, there is a need for continuous evaluation of patients' capacity to understand the information given to them.

Conclusions

With regard to defense of individuals' rights, Mediterranean ethics are ideally a synthesis of civic humanism and liberalism, incorporating the spirit of

Greek democracy, the spirit of the Enlightenment, and the achievements of the nineteenth and twentieth centuries. In Mediterranean ethics, liberalism is joined with the principles of the social welfare state.

In present-day bioethics, especially in European countries, the attempt is made to integrate both traditions—the ethics of virtues and the ethics of principles—and to go beyond adding and integrating a social element. This approach is based on the principle of solidarity and distributive justice (equity). Individual autonomy and independence of the individual from society are not proclaimed as ethical ideals, but the interdependence of persons and of nations is so proclaimed, as are, in the case of health care, greater parity and better management of resources.

A language is being developed for bioethics in Europe, and an effort is being made to determine which are the more important ethical problems in each of the European countries (see, for example, Koch et al. 1996).

References

American Psychiatric Association: Diagnostic and Statistical Manual of Mental Disorders, 4th Edition. Washington, DC, American Psychiatric Association, 1994

Aristotle: Ética a Nicómaco. Translated and notated by Bonet JP. Introduction by Íñigo EL. Madrid, Gredos, 1990

Bakan D: Freud et la tradition mystique juive. Paris, Payot, 1964

Barcia D: Necesidad de una medicina antropológica. Murcia, Spain, Publicaciones de la Universidad de Murcia, 1979

Barcia D: Ética y retraso mental: el derecho a vivir de los infradotados. Folia Humanística 30, 1992

Barcia D, Crespo MD: La relación médico-enfermo en el marco de la medicina de enlace. Actas Luso Esp Neurol Psiquiatr Cienc Afines 26 (suppl 2), 1998

Beauchamp TL, McCullough L: Ética médica. Barcelona, Labor, 1987

Becker E: La estructura del mal: un ensayo sobre la unificación de la ciencia del hombre. México City, Fondo de Cultura Económica, 1980

Blankenburg W: Zur Differentialphänomenologie der Wahnwahrnehmung: eine Studie über abnormes Bedeutungserleben. Nervenarzt 36:285–298, 1965

Braceland FJ: Historical perspectives of the ethical practice of psychiatry. Am J Psychiatry 126:230–237, 1969

Callahan P: What Kind of Life. New York, Simon & Schuster, 1991

Clouser KD: Medical ethics: some uses, abuses and limitations. N Engl J Med 293: 384–387, 1973

Crawshaw R: Greed. BMJ 313:1596–1597, 1996

Crawshaw R, Rogers DE, Pellegrino ED, et al: Patient-physician covenant. JAMA 273:1553, 1995

Elósegui M: Revindicación de la ética mediterránea como síntesis integradora de la dialectica entre éticas de la virtud y éticas de los principios. Cuadernos de Psicoética 3:474–491, 1998

Ferrater Mora J: Diccionario de filosofía, 60th Edition. Madrid, Alianza, 1979

Gafo J: Los códigos médicos, in Dilemas éticos de la medicina actual. Edited by Gafo J. Madrid, Universidad Pontificia de Comillas, 1986, pp 17–41

Gaylin W: The patient's bill of rights, in Contemporary Issues in Bioethics. Edited by Beauchamp TL, Walters L. Encino, CA, Dickenson, 1978

Gracia D: Los derechos de los enfermos, in Dilemas éticos de la medicina actual. Edited by Gafo J. Madrid, Universidad Pontificia de Comillas, 1986, pp 43–87

Gracia D: Procedimientos de decisión en ética clínica. Madrid, Endema, 1991

Gracia D, Jonsen AR: La bioética mediterranea: diálogo con la bioética americana. Diario Médico, October 23, 1998, pp 10–11

Gruhle HW: Psychologie der Schizophrenie. Berlin, Springer, 1929

Heidegger M: Sein und Zeit, 70th Edition. Tübingen, Niemeyer, 1953

Hillman J: On paranoia. Eranos 54:269–324, 1985

Jaspers K: Psicopatología general. Buenos Aires, Beta, 1955

Kilner JF: Who Lives? Who Dies? Ethical Criteria in Patient Selection. New Haven, CT, Yale University Press, 1992

Koch HG, Reiter-Theil S, Helmchen H (eds): Informed Consent in Psychiatry: European Perspectives of Ethics, Law and Clinical Practice (Medizin in Recht und Ethik, Vol 33). Baden-Baden, Nomos, 1996

Kramer PD: Listening to Prozac. New York, Viking, 1993

Kuhn R: Daseinanalyse und Psychiatrie, in Psychiatrie der Gegenwart, Vol I/2. Edited by Gruhle H. Berlin, Springer, 1963, pp 853–902

Kunz H: Zur Frage nach dem Wesen der Norm. Psyche 8:241, 321, 1954–1955

Lain Entralgo P: La relación médico-enfermo. La Revista de Occidente, March 1984

López-Ibor JJ Jr: Freud y sus ocultos dioses. Barcelona, Planeta, 1975

López-Ibor JJ Jr: Psychiatric care under the present economic era: an international perspective. European Psychiatry 12 (suppl 2):88–91, 1997

López-Ibor JJ Jr, Crespo Hervás MD: Informed consent in Spain, in Informed Consent in Psychiatry: European Perspectives of Ethics, Law and Clinical Practice (Medizin in Recht und Ethik, Vol 33). Edited by Koch HG, Reiter-Theil S, Helmchen H. Baden-Baden, Nomos, 1996, pp 233–247

López Ibor JJ Sr: La Aventura Humana. Madrid, Rialp, 1965

Marcel G: Être et avoir. Paris, Montaigne, 1955

Merleau-Ponty J: Phénoménologie de la perception. Paris, NRF Gallimard, 1945

Schneider K: Zum Begriff des Wahns. Fortschr Neurol Psychiatr 17:26–39, 1963

Vintró E: Hipócrates y la nosología hipocrática. Barcelona, Ariel, 1972

World Health Organization: International Classification of Diseases, 10th Revision. Geneva, World Health Organization, 1992

Zarader M: La dette impensée: Heidegger et l'héritage hébraïque. Paris, Seuil, 1990

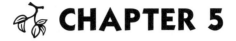 CHAPTER 5

Scandinavian Approaches

Dr. Marianne Kastrup

The former World Health Organization director General H. Nakajima (1996) wrote that "in all cultures, the people with special knowledge and powers to deal with suffering and death also have special obligations. . . . For more than a millennium in the Western medical tradition, the Hippocratic Oath has encapsulated some of the principles that are still seen as essential for good practice in the health professions. . . . Ethics, today, is a matter of lively public interest" (p. 3).

This statement reflects the increasing recognition and awareness of ethical aspects of the medical profession, both within and outside the World Health Organization, by health professionals, patients, political bodies, and the general public.

The following are pertinent questions in the present-day debate (Nakajima 1996):

- How do we strike the proper balance between the individualistic approach with a demand for services and the societal need to limit health care resources?
- How can we ensure an equitable distribution of resources to all those who need them?
- How can we ensure that the patient-doctor relationship is based on mutual respect and trust and that the two individuals see each other as partners?
- To what extent should the need for self-determination be adjusted, taking into consideration the cultural context and the need of the family?

♦ What is the future role of the doctor, when the former medical authority is lost?

♦ In this era of managed care and increasing commercialization of medicine, how do we assure respect for human values and dignity?

♦ With today's increasing bureaucratization and economic consideration of health care, how do we ensure that purely economic considerations will not override patients' interests?

With increased globalization, modern medicine and psychiatry face the same problems worldwide, and "the moral need for equality is made all the more unattainable if priority is given to progress over fairness, more over enough, and infinite goals over limited, achievable goals" (Callahan 1996, p. 8).

Although the medical profession has always been guided by a set of principles and moral codes, in the last decades there has been increasing recognition of the role of ethics in medical work. According to Barcia and Pozo (1991), the most important reasons for this situation are the technical advances in medicine, the profound secularization that has occurred recently in society and consequently also in medicine, the increasing pluralism in most Western countries with the emergence of a diversity of ideologies in society as a whole as well as in the medical field, and the increasing emphasis on and respect for the autonomy of the individual, which has altered the patient-doctor relationship.

Parallel to and as a natural consequence of these changes has been the development of a number of medical codes in general, and psychiatric codes in particular, that guide the conduct of psychiatrists. That same development has taken place in Scandinavia (in this chapter, *Scandinavia* refers to Denmark, Norway, and Sweden). In fact, there has been a long tradition in the Scandinavian countries of dealing with human rights issues, and these issues are still high on the political agenda.

This chapter is an overview of the common sociocultural features of the Scandinavian countries, the organization of the mental health care delivery systems, and the development and status of medical ethics. Also considered, with particular reference to Denmark, is how this overall cultural and ethical context is reflected in the regulations guiding the practice of psychiatrists. I discuss the local implementation of the Declaration of Madrid (reproduced in the Appendix to this book), local ethical and intercollegial regulations, and concerns regarding the achievement of ethical standards in clinical practices. I outline some of the pertinent issues in the current ethical debate, including access to medical records and medical confidentiality, patient autonomy, and collaboration with industry. Finally, I emphasize the need for psychiatrists not only to be concerned with treatment of individual patients but also to recognize their responsibility as citizens of the world.

Scandinavian Contributions to Human Rights

The medical profession in Scandinavia has contributed to the field of human rights in a number of ways. Danish physician Jens Daugaard played an important role in the development of the World Medical Association's Declaration of Tokyo (1975). The Swedish psychiatrist Clarence Blomquist was one of the creators of the Declaration of Hawaii (World Medical Association 1977). The Norwegian Medical Association established a committee on human rights that has contributed significantly in creating a forum for peaceful cooperation with and among the medical associations in the former Yugoslavia.

The first medical group of Amnesty International was founded in Denmark in 1974. Among the founders was the Danish neurologist Inge Genefke, who became one of the pioneers in medical work in the area of torture. The Danish Medical Group of Amnesty International is the only medical group that specifically focuses on medical work against the death penalty.

Characteristics of Scandinavian Countries

Common Features

The Scandinavian countries have a number of features in common. Of particular interest are the following:

Demographically, Sweden is the largest Scandinavian country, covering 450,000 square kilometers and having a population of approximately 8.5 million. Norway covers 324,000 square kilometers and has a population of 4.2 million, and Denmark has an area of 43,000 square kilometers and a population of about 5.1 million.

Collaboration between the countries is extensive and is based on a century-old feeling of having the same cultural background. This common cultural identity may be due partly to the fact that the languages of the three countries all stem from a common language, Old Nordic, and that until recently, all inhabitants of the Scandinavian countries could communicate with one another, speaking their native languages. The countries have undergone the same religious development and have established similar principles for conception of law and legislation. Collaboration is close not only in many cultural areas and in areas of research but also in areas of communication, social politics, economics, and legislation.

The Scandinavian countries have value systems that stress solidarity and justice, and the health care systems all involve a high level of public responsibility for financing and supervision. Health care financing under the taxation system (i.e., public taxes) is based on solidarity, with a balance between control by central authorities and regional responsibility for running the health care system (Holmberg 1997).

Each of the countries is a monarchy with a century-long democratic tradition. In all three countries, several political parties are represented in parliament, and coalition governments are not uncommon. There is a tradition of a high percentage of the population voting in general parliament elections and a lesser percentage voting in local elections.

All of the countries are described as welfare societies. This tradition is due to a great extent to social democratic governments' having been in power for long periods. The infrastructure, such as the public transportation system, is well developed and services are easily accessible. Characteristics of the welfare society differ from country to country but include features such as free education at the primary and secondary school levels and free and fairly easy access to higher education, which is almost exclusively public.

Health services, both primary and secondary care, are almost entirely free, with easy access to services, a very limited private health sector, and emphasis on prophylactic health care. Almost all of the extensive social services and benefits are provided in the public sector; there is little tradition of private charity, including charity for services for the elderly.

Each country has a long tradition of strong labor unions, with a high percentage of the labor force being members of unions and well-developed legislation protecting the labor force. An equally high emphasis is placed on legislation related to the protection of the physical environment.

In all Scandinavian countries, women have had a strong position traditionally, and a high percentage of women are employed full-time. There is easy access to contraception and abortion and consequently a low birth rate. A high proportion of children attend nurseries or kindergartens.

Protestantism is the state religion in all of the Scandinavian countries, but great proportions of the population are little involved in the church.

The population of each Scandinavian country is fairly homogeneous, with no long-standing tradition of integrating new and foreign ethnic groups. On the other hand, there are high mobility within the Scandinavian countries, a high degree of intermarriage among Scandinavians, and extensive possibilities of transferring educational credentials from one country to another.

Mental Health Care

In the Scandinavian countries, development in mental health care has been more or less similar, but the rate of progress has differed. Denmark was the first to establish psychiatric services in general hospitals, whereas sectorization was first implemented in Norway (Sandlund 1998).

The main trends in this region closely resemble those in many other Western countries. Inpatient care has been replaced to a large extent by community mental health services. The number of beds for psychiatric patients has been decreasing, and various kinds of support systems have been established in communities. Deinstitutionalization has also resulted in the development of a variety of other approaches (Sandlund 1998), such as multidisciplinary outpatient teams, and a range of social psychiatric interventions such as day centers and differentiated living facilities. Services are sectorized: psychiatric care is organized in such a way that a given organization with a well-defined set of services has the responsibility for the mental health services for a given geographically defined catchment area.

The provision and organization of mental health services vary to some extent from one country to another. Research projects on service provision (Sandlund 1998) clearly demonstrate that despite commonalities, the Scandinavian countries vary with respect to such aspects as numbers of beds for psychiatric patients per inhabitant and models of care provided.

Further characteristics include increased emphasis on patient autonomy and recognition of the burden carried by families of psychotic patients.

Medical Ethics

In all Scandinavian countries, ethical codes for the medical profession have a long tradition and ethical guidelines for physicians' clinical work are provided by the medical associations. Since the beginning of the 1970s, medical ethics has been taught in all Scandinavian medical schools. There is, however, no agreement about the requirement, but efforts have been made to institute uniform compulsory teaching of medical ethics in all medical schools, and in all Scandinavian countries the teaching of medical ethics at the graduate as well as the postgraduate level has been strengthened.

All Scandinavian countries have also established research ethics committees for reviewing biomedical research. These committees have been in existence for 25–30 years, and their workload is increasing, as is the number of requests for assessment of ethical aspects of individual research projects. In Denmark, the research ethics committee became legally required in 1992, and to be approved, a research protocol should include a description of the ethical aspects according to the Helsinki II Declaration (Adserballe 1997).

Scandinavian governments have recognized that there is a need for another type of ethics committee, one that does not focus on the individual research project but instead provides expertise to the government or other authorities. Such committees or ethics councils, with their composition of experts with medical, judicial, philosophical, or other relevant expertise, may also contribute to the public debate regarding issues of ethical importance. The first committee was the National Council of Medical Ethics, which was established in 1985 by the Swedish government. This committee was followed by similar committees in the other Scandinavian countries.

Within the medical associations, ethics committees have been established in all Scandinavian countries. The Danish Ethics Committee, created in 1969, was the first. These committees generally deal with topics of an ethical nature and typically include members with psychiatric expertise. Ethics committees meet on a regular basis to create ethical guidelines that are jointly agreed on or to discuss pertinent ethical topics.

Forensic Psychiatry

Despite the fact that the Scandinavian countries share the same views with respect to persons with mental illness, legislation is not identical when it comes to mental health. A number of differences are to be found in the area of forensic psychiatry (Holmberg 1997), including differences in criteria for eligibility for psychiatric treatment, extent of court involvement, the range of applicable measures, investigation of procedures, and the organization of forensic psychiatric services.

For example, in Denmark, a forensic psychiatric investigation is undertaken whenever it is likely that the findings will influence the verdict of the court. In Sweden, on the other hand, the reason for a forensic investigation is to assess whether the person committing the crime had a severe mental disorder; and in Norway, an investigation is performed to permit determination of whether the person's mental status at the time of the crime may have influenced his or her capacity to understand and control his or her actions (Holmberg 1997).

We also see differences in the mental health legislation among the Scandinavian countries. With regard to involuntary commitment, criteria are broader in Sweden than in Denmark, and commitment rates are much higher in Sweden. In Norway, commitment rates are somewhat higher than in Denmark, but the two countries have similar criteria (Engberg 1997). This means that the registration figures for involuntary commitment may reflect different patient populations and that there are various possibilities for involuntarily detaining patients who were originally admitted on a voluntary basis.

The Scandinavian countries all apply the same overall principles concerning forensic psychiatric research, namely those of autonomy (the right to make decisions about one's own life and actions), nonmaleficence (not doing harm, or minimizing harm), beneficence (doing good and eliminating suffering), and justice (equal treatment for all) (Holmberg 1997).

Psychiatric Ethics in Denmark

In this section, the focus is not on the Scandinavian countries in general but on Denmark in particular. Several guidelines and codes regulate the work of psychiatrists in Denmark.

Ethical and Intercollegial Regulations

The Danish Medical Association developed ethical and intercollegial regulations, the latest revision of which was adopted by the Assembly of Representatives in 1989 (Danish Medical Association 1989). These regulations have the purpose of strengthening good medical practice and confidence and cooperation between doctors and patients (Section 1). They deal with the doctor's obligation to work for the prevention of illness and the enhancement of health, acting in a careful and conscientious manner and to the best of his or her ability to relieve pain and help sick patients to regain health. While the doctor does this, the dignity and personal integrity of the patient should be respected (Section 2).

The doctor is required to treat according to the highest standards with regard to the given condition (Section 3). The patient has the right "to full information about diagnosis, prognosis and treatment possibilities. Further . . . the doctor always must to the best of his or her ability identify with the patient's overall psychological, social, and somatic situation, and carefully consider the spirit in which information should be given. Thus, the doctor ought not force information on a patient who clearly does not want it" (Section 4; Danish Medical Association 1989)

The importance of professional secrecy is stated in Section 5, which emphasizes the patient's right to discretion even after the death of the patient, unless the patient has given his or her consent for disclosure of the information. When legislation obligates a doctor to make a statement to a public authority about the patient's health or personal affairs, the information given must be restricted to only that which is absolutely necessary to process the specific case. Aside from this, a doctor may disclose health and personal information about a patient only when doing so is essential for the good of the patient or to save the lives of others or repudiate evidently false allegations.

Doctors can participate in the establishment of registers of patients or human research subjects only when they take full responsibility (Section 6). Further, a doctor who enters into cooperation with laypersons treating patients assumes responsibility for the diagnosis and treatment (Section 7). The obligation to act is presented in Section 8, which states that when a doctor is summoned to a sick person and the information received indicates that immediate medical help is necessary, he or she must render this assistance as soon as possible.

A doctor ought to publicize any research result of significance and present it at a medical forum before communicating it to the public (Section 9). If a doctor speaks as a representative of an association or a public or private establishment, the capacity in which he or she is speaking must be indicated (Section 10).

Doctors need to participate in the debate about health policy issues (Section 11). The most essential content of the Declaration of Tokyo and the Nordic Medical Association's statements against doctors' participation in capital punishment is presented in Section 12. The obligations in connection with biomedical research with respect to informed consent, involving reporting to regional scientific ethics committees, are stated in Section 13.

Recording of identifiable patients for educational purposes or in connection with information-related activities may take place only with the consent of those concerned, and it is the doctor's responsibility that the use of recording be in accordance with good medical practice (Section 14).

Doctors should be hindered from participation in screening of the labor force for the labor market (Section 15), unless such participation is required by legislation or is supported by urgent needs of the patient or others. A doctor taking part in a collective labor action is still bound by his or her ethical obligations, but doctors like all other wage earners have the right to strike (Section 16).

Finally, a doctor may in no way cooperate with the advertising or marketing of projects injurious to health (Section 17) and should exercise care that statements about health research are not composed in such a manner that they could be construed as advertisements.

These ethical regulations govern the practice of Danish doctors. One need not be a member of the Danish Medical Association to work as a physician in Denmark; the authorization to work as a physician is issued by the National Board of Health, a government body. However, only a very small number of doctors are not members of the association. It should be mentioned that the country has no medical council that monitors the behavior of individual doctors, but the Danish Medical Association has an ethics board that deals with complaints about individual doctors' behavior.

Membership for Danish psychiatrists in the Danish Psychiatric Association, a scientific society, is also voluntary. The Danish Psychiatric Association has not developed its own ethical codes or guidelines but adheres to the ethical codes of the Danish Medical Association and the Declaration of Madrid.

The Declaration of Madrid

In 1996, the General Assembly of the World Psychiatric Association adopted the Declaration of Madrid. Subsequently, the Declaration of Madrid became known to Danish psychiatrists, but no full Danish translation exists.

Article 1 of the declaration, outlining the role of psychiatry, fits well into the Danish setting. In particular, the statement that "psychiatrists should be aware of and concerned with the equitable allocation of health resources" is in line with the Danish public health system's providing free and easy access to mental health care for all inhabitants.

In Article 2, it is mentioned that "psychiatrists trained in research should seek to advance the scientific frontiers of psychiatry." There is a long-standing tradition in Denmark of involving physicians in medical research during their specialty training, and the introduction of a research certificate as part of postgraduate training has been discussed by the Research Committee of the Danish Psychiatric Association. Any research undertaken is carried out under the supervision of an experienced colleague and requires approval by the regional research ethics committee.

Article 3, allowing a patient to make free and informed decisions, is in accordance with Danish practice and concern for patient autonomy.

Article 4 deals with the problem of treatment against a patient's will. Such treatment is also discussed in Article 12 of the Danish Mental Health Act of 1989 (Law No. 331). There it is stated that treatment against a patient's will is only possible for persons who are psychotic and are dangerous to themselves or others or for persons who are psychotic and who would be less likely to be cured or to improve if they were not treated.

Forced treatment typically involves administration of medication, and the use of depot neuroleptics should be avoided. The patient may complain about the decision to administer medication, and unless treatment is a matter of life or death, the psychiatrist cannot proceed before the patient board of appeal, to which the patient has complained, has approved the doctor's decision.

The Mental Health Act also permits treatment of a physical illness against a patient's will. For such treatment to be given, the patient should meet the same criteria as discussed earlier.

Article 5 of the Declaration of Madrid, on assessment of patients and third-party situations, is well in accordance with current forensic psychiatric practice in Denmark.

Article 6 deals with confidentiality. The wording of Article 6 gives rise to no problems, but it is currently a matter of concern in Denmark that medical confidentiality is increasingly being challenged by third parties with an interest in the history and condition of the patient in question. Thus, a patient may give informed consent for a third party (e.g., an insurance company) to receive detailed information about the patient's psychiatric history; such consent may be a requirement to obtain an insurance policy.

In Article 7, on psychiatric research activities, a comment refers to the fact that junior psychiatrists under proper supervision are involved in research activities, but the article also states that all research protocols should be sent for approval to regional research ethics committees.

The guidelines concerning specific situations, in the Declaration of Madrid, are in accordance with current Danish practice:

- *Euthanasia.* This guideline emphasizes the particular problems related to a distorted view due to mental illness. According to Danish legislation, no doctor can participate in euthanasia.
- *Torture.* The statement that psychiatrists should not take part in torture is reflected in the leading role that Danish physicians have played in the medical work against torture.
- *Death penalty.* In 1986, the Nordic Medical Association took a strong stand against doctors' participating directly or indirectly in administration of the death penalty. The death penalty has been abolished in all Scandinavian countries.
- *Selection of sex.* Termination of pregnancy because of the sex of the fetus is not an issue of concern in Denmark.
- *Organ transplantation.* The recommendation of this specific guideline is in accordance with Danish practice.

The Danish Mental Health Act

The Danish Mental Health Act (Law No. 331 of May 24, 1989; revised June 14, 1995 in Law Nos. 386 and 389) states that any admission to and treatment in a psychiatric institution must take place with the patient's consent, if at all possible, and that the psychiatrist should inform the patient about the purpose of the admission and treatment as well as the prognosis of his or her condition.

In the most recent revision of the Mental Health Act, the concept of the treatment plan was introduced. The psychiatrist responsible for a given treatment is also responsible for the development of a treatment plan for any person admitted and must advise the patient about the content of the plan and seek the patient's consent for its implementation. The treatment plan must be comprehensive: it must include psychopathological, somatic, and social aspects; information on the patient's acceptance of the plan; and the time of evaluation of the treatment plan. The treatment plan has turned out to be a useful instrument in the modern multidisciplinary psychiatric setting, and it may be seen as useful for making explicit the goals of the therapeutic interventions proposed and the patient's consent thereto (Adserballe 1997).

The Mental Health Act deals with conditions of involuntary admission and criteria to be fulfilled in the case of treatment against a patient's will. An overall principle guiding the Mental Health Act is the principle of minimal means. An innovative part of the Mental Health Act is the introduction of patient counselors, who are employed by the county and are independent of the psychiatric institution in the area. In the case of use of any force, whether related to admission, discharge, or treatment, the psychiatric patient is assigned a patient counselor whose main function is to guide the patient with respect to all conditions related to admission, stay, and treatment on the psychiatric ward. The counselor may also help the patient in the case of a complaint. Patient counselors may be seen as a body that monitors the use of force in psychiatric institutions, a body that has access to all documents related thereto.

Article 2 of the Mental Health Act states that to prevent the use of force, the health authority should offer care and treatment of "good hospital standard." This phrase is a result (though meager) of extensive lobbying while the Mental Health Act was in preparation. Part of the committee preparing the act proposed, being strongly supported by psychiatrists, that the legislation be very specific and include minimum requirements with regard to patients such as 1 hour per day in the open air, private rooms, acceptable room standards, and access to meaningful activities and education. This ethical challenge to ensure minimum requirements was overridden by economic concerns and a reluctance to give precise standards and norms for services (Adserballe 1997).

Finally, it should be mentioned that the Danish Mental Health Act clearly refers only to persons who are psychotic or the equivalent. Persons with alcohol or drug abuse problems are not affected by the legislation unless they are psychotic.

In a recent publication by the Ethics Council (Etisk Råd 1996), it was again brought forward that future legislation should be more specific in terms of minimum rules for services provided for psychiatric patients. The following year, the Ethics Council (Etisk Råd 1997) recommended that psychiatric patients admitted have private rooms, live in modern, homelike facilities, have access to meaningful activities and education, have a minimum of 1 hour per day outdoors, and, according to need, have the opportunity for accompanied leave.

It is proposed that these conditions be granted to all psychiatric patients admitted. The Ethics Council also found it worth considering that a psychiatric patient could declare on admission what kinds of treatment would be acceptable if he or she should later become unable to act rationally.

Doctors at Risk

The Ethics Committee of the Danish Medical Association pointed out the particular ethical problems with which so-called doctors at risk are faced (Adserballe 1997). Doctors at risk are medical doctors who may be employed by nonmedical authorities and who have tasks and duties other than the traditional therapeutic ones. Military doctors, prison doctors, forensic psychiatrists, and forensic scientists may fall into this category. Psychiatrists working in penitentiaries may be faced with ethical dilemmas, conflicts between the interest of the patient and that of the judicial system. The Danish Medical Association has always taken a strong stand against legitimizing coercive interventions by the judicial system, such as solitary confinement. The sole concern of the medical doctor is to diagnose and treat disorders.

Objectives for Quality in Psychiatric Care

An expert committee appointed by the Danish National Board of Health outlined the objectives for quality in psychiatric care (Sundhedsstyrelsen 1995). The report stemmed from the fact that mental health care has undergone an extensive reorganization, leading toward decentralization, over the last decade; that as a consequence of this reorganization, psychiatry and other medical disciplines no longer belong to the same health authority in some regions; that development of diagnostic and treatment methods in psychiatry continues; that as a result of this development, there is specialization in treatment of particular groups of psychiatric patients; and that there is increasing public interest in the quality of the mental health care.

The report provides a comprehensive view of the objectives with respect to referral for care, diagnosis and assessment, treatment, discharge, and rehabilitation. The report may be described as pragmatic with a realistic approach to standards of care. On the other hand, little attention is paid in this report to the ethical dimensions of psychiatric care. Also, the focus is on national aspects and there is no discussion of the global challenges faced by psychiatrists today.

The Ethical Perspective

The Ethics Council (Etisk Råd 1996) outlined the objectives for psychiatric intervention in Denmark, and the focus under the heading "The Ethical Perspective" in the report is on two areas of intervention: prevention, treatment, and care of symptoms; and improvement of the quality of life of mentally ill patients and of their opportunities to lead fulfilling lives. The Ethics Council called for more dialogue between patients, relatives, psychiatrists, other mental health professionals, politicians, and others to determine priorities.

The Ethics Council listed five ideals:

1. *Care of patients with mental illness.* Society has a duty to ensure necessary treatment for mentally ill individuals, a central principle in the Danish welfare model, according to which all in need of care should be treated adequately.
2. *Respect for the dignity and integrity of mentally ill persons.* Individuals with mental illness, like any other individuals, have the right to be respectfully treated even though they may, in some situations, be unable to act rationally. Respect for a person's integrity implies a respect for the value of the person's experiences (Etisk Råd 1996) and, in the Danish context, the granting of the opportunity to be alone.
3. *Respect for the autonomy of patients with mental illness.* In the debate in Denmark, there is an increasing emphasis on individual autonomy and the patient's right to make decisions regarding treatment and care.
4. *Protection of others against violations by mentally ill patients.* With the deinstitutionalization of psychiatric care, there has been an increase in the number of mentally ill patients living isolated in the community. Increased interaction between persons with mental illness and the general public has resulted, and many people may feel threatened or insecure when faced with a mentally ill person.
5. *Security against abuse of psychiatry.* The fact that psychiatry, contrary to other medical disciplines, provides an opportunity to use force necessi-

tates a close regulation of psychiatric practice (Etisk Råd 1996). Of particular concern for many is the possibility, as evidenced in the Danish Mental Health Act, that patients who are voluntarily admitted may be detained against their will. This can occur if psychiatrists consider such patients psychotic and in immediate danger to themselves or others or if it is believed that discharge (i.e., no treatment) would result in significant deterioration of health.

Issues of Concern

Several issues with an ethical dimension confront Danish psychiatrists apart from the areas outlined in the Mental Health Act. Some of these issues are discussed here.

Access to Medical Records

Danish patients have had access to their hospital records since 1987 and to the records of other health professionals since 1994. Many psychiatrists have expressed concern over patient access to patient records because mentally ill persons may find it problematic to be confronted with their own histories. This access appears to have given rise to a few problems. Nowadays, psychiatric patients frequently request access to their personal files and may either be given photocopies or meet with their psychiatrists to go through the files. A positive consequence of this access legislation has been that psychiatrists abstain from writing personal comments of a prejudicial nature. It is not customary to have a double filing system, with one official medical file and unofficial notes kept out of reach of the patient. Once again, psychiatrists have been faced with the fact that psychiatric patients have a lot of common sense and quite a realistic approach to their own conditions. Few Danish psychiatrists today consider it an ethical problem to give their patients full access to all of the medical information.

Medical Confidentiality

The Ethics Regulations of the Danish Medical Association as well as the Declaration of Madrid emphasize the doctor's duty to keep in confidence all information obtained in the therapeutic context. Medical information may be handed from one doctor to another within the same administrative authority without the consent of the patient. On the other hand, a psychiatrist (or any other hospital doctor) is no longer allowed to provide the primary care physician in charge of follow-up treatment the relevant psychiatric information without patient consent.

In two recent Danish court cases, psychiatrists who had not maintained medical confidentiality, acting in what they thought was their patients' best interest, were sued by their patients.

There is, however, increasing concern in the Danish medical profession that other interests may override medical confidentiality. Thus, if a patient wants to obtain certain benefits from social services, he or she cannot refuse to provide relevant medical information on his or her particular case. Similarly, it is not possible to obtain a public pension unless relevant medical information is provided. Furthermore, in criminal cases, courts can order that relevant medical information be released.

Relatives of psychiatric patients frequently express dissatisfaction with the interpretation by psychiatrists of confidentiality. The psychiatrist considers himself or herself the patient's advocate, which means that the spouse and parents may be unable to obtain any information about the condition of the patient, determine whether the patient is receiving proper care, or learn what the future plans are, without the approval of the patient. In daily hospital practice, confidentiality is frequently maintained in a rather inflexible way, to the extent that a relative contacting a ward may be unable to obtain any information on the patient's condition. Currently, there is an increasing recognition among psychiatrists that protection of patients' rights vis-à-vis the interest of relatives has gone too far in many instances and that such a situation is not in the best interest of the patient.

Patient Autonomy

Closely related to medical confidentiality is patient autonomy. Emphasis on autonomy is part of Scandinavian culture, and, as pointed out by the Ethics Council (Etisk Råd 1996), lack of autonomy is considered the greatest unhappiness of the modern person, and consequently the ultimate goal of all treatment for mentally ill patients is the regaining of autonomy. The ideal is to be able to organize life in a rational manner and to live independently, without the need for support from others.

The key role of patient autonomy has been increasingly emphasized in recent years. A patient has the right to make decisions about his or her treatment without interference from family or health professionals. In this context, an alliance between the doctor and the patient's family seems meaningless, given that present legislation clearly states that informed consent is the key principle in all treatment, with the exception of situations outlined in the Mental Health Act.

The balance between a paternalistic approach and respect for patient autonomy is delicate, not least in the case of psychiatric patients, whose mental conditions may render them temporarily unable to exercise judgment. To provide care for those who are suffering is part of a doctor's duty. The 1948 Declaration of Geneva (World Medical Association 1970) states: "The health of my patient shall be my first consideration." That is, the autonomy of the patient is not of first importance. Tranøy (1991) suggested that to solve this dilemma, a distinction be made between strong and weak paternalism. It may be ethically acceptable to interfere with a person's autonomy when doing so will be in the patient's best interest (strong paternalism). On the other hand, it may be ethically acceptable to interfere with a person's autonomy if that person lacks information or is otherwise not competent to make informed choices (weak paternalism). In the case of psychiatric care, the latter situation may be relevant.

Ethical problems relate to the political agenda that citizens have a responsibility for the quality of their own lives and for their own health. This may sound convincing and in line with the cultural focus on individual autonomy, but this approach—that the individual is responsible for his or her own state of health—is a double-edged sword (Kastrup 1992). It may be that groups of human beings who do not exhibit the correct health-promoting behavior and proper life management seemingly lack sufficient motivation to remain healthy and as a consequence may experience a subsequent lack of treatment resources. Psychiatric patients are among the losers in this game.

Hunger Strikes

Hunger strikes represent a particular problem in the area of patient autonomy. What is considered correct medical behavior toward a person on a hunger strike has changed in recent years from more paternalistic behavior to an approach based on patient autonomy (Holmberg 1997). The 1975 Declaration of Tokyo states that a prisoner who is capable of rational judgment and refuses nourishment should not be fed artificially. Up to 1992, the Danish National Board of Health was of the opinion that prisoners on hunger strikes should be transferred to the hospital and treated if they became unconscious. Today the National Board of Health has changed its recommendation, which is in line with that of the World Medical Association. In practice, it is the psychiatrists working in the Danish penitentiary system who are faced with the problem of assessing the competence of those on hunger strikes and dealing with the subsequent ethical dilemma if the hunger strikes continue.

Collaboration Between the Medical Profession and Industry

The importance of independence of the medical profession from external economic interests is recognized both by the Danish Psychiatric Association and the Danish Medical Association. Both organizations emphasize the necessity for clear guidelines on sponsorship. The guidelines approved by the Medical Association in 1993 and 1994 are public and may help psychiatrists to act ethically with regard to gifts, economic privileges, benefits for traveling companions, and other financial temptations.

Similarly, guidelines were approved by the Danish Medical Association in 1994 regarding clinical trials. There it was again emphasized that the medical profession and the drug industry must remain clearly independent and that regulations for good clinical practice must be respected in all clinical trials.

Conclusions

We as psychiatrists are faced with two ethical challenges (Kastrup 1991). One has to do with how we as individuals manage situations in our daily clinical practices that require personal ethical decisions. Pertinent issues in the debate about psychiatry in Denmark are primarily local and related to the provision of mental health care and aspects of that care, such as the advantages and shortcomings of community mental health care, the number of beds available for psychiatric patients, and the division of responsibility between health services and social services with respect to social psychiatric interventions.

The other ethical challenge has to do with how we as citizens, not only of our own countries but of the world, contribute to an ethically acceptable, more equitable allocation of the resources available for mental health care (Kastrup 1991). We have a long way to go to achieve fair distribution.

Today, little attention is paid to the fact that the Baltic countries are faced with severe problems with respect to mental health care. Furthermore, not many psychiatrists ask how Danish psychiatrists may provide assistance to other parts of the world in greater need of care and with shortages of resources. Becoming aware of our common problems, irrespective of culture, and recognizing the importance of establishing professional networks across regions are not yet high on the agenda of psychiatrists.

It is interesting that the first reaction of my department when I, having returned from the X World Congress of Psychiatry, reported on the newly adopted Declaration of Madrid was to ask "What effect will this have on our own psychiatry department?" Let this be an event of the past.

References

Adserballe H: Etik i psykiatrien. Copenhagen, Munksgaard, 1997

Barcia D, Pozo P: Ethical aspects of psychiatry, in The European Handbook of Psychiatry and Mental Health. Edited by Seva A. Saragossa, Spain, Antropos, 1991, pp 2277–2294

Callahan D: Achievable goals. World Health 5:6–8, 1996

Danish Medical Association: Ethical and Inter-collegial Regulations. Copenhagen, Danish Medical Association, 1989

Danish Mental Health Act (Act on Detention and Other Coercive Measures in Psychiatry). May 24, 1989 (Law No. 331). Revised June 14, 1995 (Law Nos. 386 and 389)

Engberg M: Investigating compulsory care—experiences from a planned study at the Nordic level. Nordic Journal of Psychiatry 51 (suppl 39):63–65, 1997

Etisk Råd: Psykiatriske patienters vilkår. Copenhagen, Etisk Råd, 1996

Etisk Råd: Psykiatriske patienters vilkår—en redegørelse. Copenhagen, Etisk Råd, 1997

Holmberg G: Forensic psychiatric practice in the Nordic countries. Nordic Journal of Psychiatry 51 (suppl 39):7–14, 1997

Kastrup M: Den etiske udfordring—psykiateren som enkeltindivid og samfundsborger, in Tvång-autonomi: etik i psykiatri (SOS-rapport 19). Stockholm, Socialstyrelsen, 1991, pp 144–150

Kastrup M: Egenomsorg—et tveægget sværd, in Psykiatri og forebyggelse. Edited by Rosenbaum B. Copenhagen, Sundhedskomiteen, 1992, pp 127–136

Nakajima H: Health, ethics and human rights (editorial). World Health 5:3, 1996

Sandlund M: A Nordic multicenter study on sectorized psychiatry (dissertation). Umeå University, Umeå, Sweden, 1998

Sundhedsstyrelsen: Målsætninger for kvalitet i voksenpsykiatrien. Copenhagen, Sundhedsstyrelsen, 1995

Tranøy KE: Tvang–autonomi–etikk, in Tvång-autonomi: etik i psykiatri (SOS-rapport 19). Stockholm, Socialstyrelsen, 1991, pp 13–19

World Medical Association: Declaration of Geneva (1948), in Declaration of Geneva; Declaration of Helsinki; Declaration of Sydney; Declaration of Oslo. New York, World Medical Association, 1970

World Medical Association: Declaration of Tokyo. New York, World Medical Association, 1975

World Medical Association: Declaration of Hawaii. New York, World Medical Association, 1977

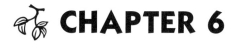 **CHAPTER 6**

Culture and Ethics of Managed Care in the United States

Dr. Renato D. Alarcon

Considered an example of an open society, the United States is a natural laboratory for the complex interactions between culture and ethics. This reality stems both from a multifaceted historical background unfolded in a relatively short period—no more than 300 years—and a complicated tapestry of psychocultural features and health-related characteristics. Such interactions are open to exploration and debate, given that the fields of mental health and psychiatric ethics are not necessarily uniform or entirely compatible. In this chapter, I examine these aspects, focusing primarily on the ethical impact of managed care against the cultural background of an always evolving American society.

Historical Outline

The arrival of the first immigrants on the coast of Massachusetts was a historical event of extraordinary proportions because it dramatized the drastic defense of religious and ethical principles as well as the search for the opportunity (and the hope) to act on them freely (Parrington 1930). The immi-

The author gratefully acknowledges the assistance of Gregory Smith, M.D., and the technical help of Ms. Terry Lawson.

grants' coexistence with the original inhabitants of the vast new continent also put to the test the endurance of such principles. Other factors such as education, group dynamics, political sophistication, and concepts of property, work, and family, together with obvious differences in complexion and other physiognomic characteristics, set the stage for confrontation. The continuous influx of new immigrants, many of them not sharing the values and cultural characteristics of the original immigrants, was palliated by the endless opening of new opportunities for property and wealth envisioned by the pioneering explorers of the West (Billington 1949). However, this process of conquest also meant actual military confrontations with the native Americans, organized by then in defense of their land and their culture. The clash of good and evil and the protection of a cultural legacy brought from Europe in the form of religion, language, education, and other concrete aspects of life collided with more abstract, nature-bound, and nature-oriented group philosophies of native tribes and close allegiance to myths and many gods (Maybury-Lewis 1992). Thus, the conquest of the West was a process of economic absorption in the name of different notions of civilization, beliefs, and ethics.

The War of Independence fought during the last quarter of the eighteenth century reaffirmed a sense of dignity and sanctioned the possibility of innovative political experiments. Yet the gradual, sometimes deliberate, elimination of native groups by means of cultural absorption, economic subjugation, or bloody military actions led to another major national issue: slavery. By the middle of the nineteenth century, America enjoyed, and was proud of, the label of "land of opportunity," a country in which individual initiative, an ethic of hard work, old-fashioned values, and continuously developing capitalistic philosophies converged as "bastions of civilization" among the "barbarian" native groups. The end justified the means, and the means were the subject of strong rationalizations sanctioned by local representatives of distant governments and imported religions—no matter how varied the latter's original sources were. Those were the initial but momentous times in which the inherent but already palpable tensions of pluralism and diversity were confronted (Trinterud 1949).

The Civil War, one of the bloodiest military confrontations in the history of the world, dealt not only with economic considerations but with the most profound ethical issues for the young nation: whether words of the Constitution and the Bill of Rights and the avowed pursuit of high moral and religious standards were true facts of American life or simple rhetoric of heroic times. Historians almost unanimously agree that although the outcome of this conflict seemed to consolidate the high ethical principles of the nation, deep wounds, divisions, distrust, and mutual recriminations remained to generate other significant realignments and historical changes in the life of the United States: the civil rights movement of the 1960s and beyond was a new chapter in this saga.

By the latter part of the nineteenth century, the United States was on the road to becoming the world's first economic superpower. The two world wars were testing grounds for the resilience of the American people, their industrial strength, and the advantages of being a country that stretched across a whole continent and was therefore almost immune to the risk of foreign invasions. Taking the lead against the Nazi regime and its racist philosophy gave the United States the moral power to exercise political leadership across the globe.

The Cold War (1948–1989) represented the ongoing confrontation of two political and economic systems that, in a different version, reproduced for both sides the conflict between good and evil. The United States considered the fight against the expansion of communism in the world as its unequivocal first priority. The implementation of this principle took forms that were dramatic (the Berlin Airlift), warring (the Korean conflict), and even extreme and bizarre (McCarthyism), culminating with an unpopular war in the jungles of Southeast Asia by the middle 1960s. America was the champion of democracy, the leader of the free world, the defender of freedom and justice, the ultimate embodiment of what was then and is even now called Western Judeo-Christian culture.

The fall of the Soviet Union in the beginning of the 1990s appeared to have created a new world order, prematurely saluted as the universal establishment of peace, freedom, democracy, justice, and progress. The United States assumed a new role, but soon the new world order was challenged by new forces. Religious fundamentalism, ethnic polarizations, regional wars, economic collapses, corruption, narcotic traffic, violence, and a number of other developments have led to changes in the United States' view of the world. A reluctant superpower, or, according to others, a superpower weary of exercising all the possibilities of a persuasive approach to world affairs, finds itself struggling with a changing cultural environment. The quiet 1950s, the thunderous 1960s, the sobering 1970s (with Watergate, the end of the Vietnam War, and the first oil-supply crisis), the uncertain 1980s, and the premillennium 1990s have all added their quotas of trials and pains, challenges and issues that test the ethical fiber of an ebullient society. The technological revolution and the conquest of cyberspace continuously shape and reshape the cultural background of America. This in itself is not new, for culture is, by definition, ever changing. Nevertheless, what some consider "eternal truths" are maintained as guiding lights in an uncertain journey. The ethics of this continuous change is perhaps the biggest challenge.

American Psychocultural Features

What are or what could be those permanent features of American culture today? Which ones are particularly close to the ethical scrutiny of social scientists and, more specifically, mental health professionals? Is it possible to identify them, or is the notion of ephemeral values more powerful than their historical weight? These are questions that have no easy answers. In this section, the main psychocultural features of contemporary American life are reviewed in an effort to describe the backdrop against which more specific health- and mental health–related factors can be examined.

The United States is a country where individual freedoms are exercised with few if any restrictions. Freedom of speech, press, religion, and work, zealously defended (and interpreted) by all kinds of people, is the hallmark of American life. Tolerance and acceptance of these freedoms is legally and institutionally sanctioned. The institutional sanctioning may be exemplified by the growing and stronger presence of women and ethnic minorities in the sometimes noisy but always healthy public debates on many issues. The pluralism almost automatically derived from the exercise of these freedoms led to the consideration of American society first as a melting pot and later as a multicultural society struggling both to preserve its basic, common tenets and to respect the uniqueness of its many components (Clark 1970).

Hard work as the basis for personal advancement, economic and financial gain, and concomitant social ascent is another factor in American life. Based on the Calvinist principle of God's rewarding the good, honest work of good Christians while they are still on earth, this cultural principle is also continuously debated, reviewed, and revised as the population deals with welfare and work issues (Weber 1930). The veneration of family as the social nucleus of progress, work, love, and preservation of values is another basic component of the American cultural fabric. Finally, the search for a balanced view of public issues, away from the extremes of the political spectrum, and the continuous debate on the benefits and flaws of such an essentially centrist position has led to what some find a rather ambiguous alternative: political compromise. From a different perspective, this may be the healthiest and least imperfect of political practices.

These debates are the result of the country's almost obsessive tendency toward self-observation and self-criticism. It is as though the objective of being better can only be predicated on the fact that one must be one's own harshest critic (Potter 1973). This leads to another characteristic of the culture of the United States: the seemingly endless pursuit of change for the sake of change. The effervescence of American life appears to fuel this trend, as does the ever-present and ever-changing technology. This sometimes confusing public debate may lead to other psychocultural features that, in some cases, look like negative images of the positive ones mentioned earlier (Walters 1978). For instance, individual freedom and the right to obtain reward for hard, well-done work have reinforced the notion of individualism (the rugged individualism of the conqueror of the West, the cowboy, the self-appointed vigilante) and the concomitant valuing of individual rights to the detriment of collective rights. The pursuit of happiness and material wealth, as well as the consecration of the market forces as the "driving engines of progress," has led to the fostering of consumerism in ways that only reinforce selfish practices (as opposed to idealism and altruism) and materialistic, money-based hierarchies (as opposed to the egalitarianism postulated by democratic principles) (Pessen 1971; Schor 1998). In the health field, the public's seemingly insatiable demand for medicines and procedures that prolong life at any price clearly reflects the same distortions.

The moral and social foundations of the family as society's nucleus are also being threatened by these forces. This explains the shaky realities of communities across the country and the struggle of these communities to define themselves in the face of changing economic and demographic factors. The frustrations of urban life, the rapid pace set in the workplace, the competitiveness that feeds the proverbial American individualism, and the tapestry of ethnic minorities in the country lead to an array of additional negative features: religious fundamentalism, breeding intolerance and ill-directed zeal, and racism in different guises or through ambiguous statements by public officials and private citizens (Carter 1995).

In summary, the face of America and, moreover, America's set of cultural values are an ever-changing, kaleidoscopic stage where the life of almost 300 million people in the richest country of the world unfolds. The nation's ethical compass is continuously tested by these realities, which have a powerful impact on the health and mental health of the American people and on the ethical bases of the professionals' work.

The Mental Health Field

American psychiatry is as pluralistic as the United States' population in contemporary times. Benjamin Rush, considered the father of American psychiatry, was among the signers of the Declaration of Independence in 1776. He epitomized the social commitment of the practitioners of the incipient specialty in America (Blain and Barton 1979). Psychiatry was the first medical specialty to be organized in a professional and scientific group, the Association of Medical Superintendents of American Institutions for the Insane, founded in 1844 (Wittels 1946). American psychiatry has been both a receptacle for contributions from many quarters and an active, creative, and innovative engine of progress through the very American ingenuity and entrepreneurial initiative. The European contributions, twists, turns, and fads were eagerly received in the New World's biggest country. Such was the case with the establishment of asylums, the early neuropsychiatric perspectives, Adolf Mayer's psychobiological school, psychoanalysis, community and social psychiatry, and more recently the predominance of biological psychiatry. How America has mostly contributed is through its spectacular technological progress, particularly in recent decades. From the use of computer programs to advances in neuroimaging, molecular genetics techniques, and the new frontiers of cognitive neuroscience, American psychiatry has attached itself to the different revolutions in psychiatry through the last 100 years (Ackerknecht 1968). Not surprisingly, and given the political power of the country, American contributions from all these quarters have literally swept the world at different times. The success of the three latest versions of the American Psychiatric Association's *Diagnostic and Statistical Manual of Mental Disorders* (DSM-III, DSM-III-R, and DSM-IV) (American Psychiatric Association 1980, 1987, 1994) is only one proof of these accomplishments (Alarcon 1995; Wilson 1993).

It is clear, however, that the quality of the mental health field in the United States does not necessarily reflect the country's leadership in technology, information science, and basic and clinical research. For once, the political process has been unable to keep in step with scientific progress. The dynamics of demographic change may help clarify some aspects of this situation. For instance, if the country's ethnic minorities become the majority within the next 25–50 years, the continuously uneven distribution of wealth may well lead to a potentially dangerous polarization. If the public and the private resources are unequally accessible and available to the different ethnic and demographic groups, the provision of adequate mental health care will suffer as a result. Some of these problems are already evident in several parts of the country.

The role of the media in the depiction of and the debate around mental health issues has not been entirely analyzed, yet their influence in shaping public opinion is undeniable. This can indeed make or break the public's views about ethnic groups, mental health and mental illness, and the fate of issues such as stereotyping and stigmatization. This unique phenomenon of the last quarter of the twentieth century will only increase in power and influence. Along the same lines, the media can help either magnify or reduce the impact of violence in American society. Unquestionably, the mental health of the American people will depend in no small part on the direction, depth, and scope of media coverage of all kinds of issues and events.

Another important component of the current scene in the United States is the role of lay groups and organizations, coalitions of relatives of mentally ill people, human rights advocates, and citizen and political organizations that have taken increasing interest in mental health and mental illness issues. Some of these groups have obtained significant political and economic lobbying power, and all add a singular dimension to the way mental illness is seen in the country. The greater visibility of mental illness owes as much to the celebrities who have come forward to talk about their emotional problems as to these organizations of concerned citizens that have taken advantage of the openness of a democratic society to advance their causes (Torrey et al. 1990).

The old debates about psychosocial versus biomedical aspects of the etiology, pathogenesis, diagnosis, and prognosis of mental illness have taken on new guises. It is undeniable, for example, that behind the rhetoric of integrated and comprehensive care, a significant struggle is taking place about whether public and private clinical and research monies should be devoted to biological and pharmacological approaches to psychiatric conditions or to the less spectacular and perhaps more laborious psychosocial, rehabilitation, and chronic care approaches. In this sense, some of the lay organizations have decidedly taken the biomedical view of mental illness, partly as a reaction to many decades of psychoanalytically inspired, guilt-ridden, and veiled (or overt) criticism of parental behavior as *the* cause of mental illness, and partly because of more statistically and experimentally demonstrable results in shorter periods, particularly for acute and early-diagnosed conditions. The ethical implications of this debate are obvious.

The stage on which all these factors display their strength is in many ways run today by the multifaceted "managed care revolution." Although its penetration in the mental health field is smaller than in other branches of medical practice, the ethical issues raised by the managed care approach are salient. The cost of psychiatric care depends on the availability and variety of services as much as on what the potential "consumer" can afford. The quality of the professionals providing care, their background, and their level of training and skill do have as many financial implications as ethical ones. Even the way in which managed care companies rank and deal with mental illness and mental health professionals reveals the respect or lack of it for these conditions, the assessment of their human and emotional cost, and the level at which mental illness stands compared with other medical conditions. The choice of treatment, length of contact, number of encounters or sessions, payment of services, and terms of the patient-therapist and the managed care organization–mental health professional relationships do have an enormous and as yet not totally explored ethical impact.

Ethical Perspectives on Psychiatric Managed Care

The result of a long series of historical, social, and cultural events in the United States, managed care is now considered not only a powerful factor in the economy, quality, and efficiency of patient care but also a fundamental challenge to the ethics of the medical profession itself. In the remainder of this chapter, I focus on such implications, attempting to dissect the issues surrounding managed care.

Review of Mental Health Care Economics

Throughout the first two centuries of their country's existence, Americans paid for their care personally, physicians' fees were the result of private negotiations with patients and their families, and the doctor-patient relationship was based almost entirely on a trust generated by moral imperatives proclaimed, sometimes stentoriously, by the profession itself. As a result, the social esteem of the medical profession grew immeasurably.

The practice of psychiatry as a specialty developed only after World War II, fostered by the impact of new intellectual, socioeconomic, and political developments. Quite significant among them were the influence of psychoanalytic tenets preached by Freud (who had a rather successful visit to the United States in 1907) and an outstanding cadre of his followers, the development of outpatient psychiatric care, the popularity of democratic principles, the beginnings of destigmatization of mental illness, and the advent and rapid growth of private insurance.

From the start, the essential purpose of medicine and psychiatry was to help, heal, and comfort sick persons and to protect them from harm. This principle, now called *beneficence*, formed the main thrust of the Hippocratic Oath. Other requirements of the physician—such as competence, confidentiality, or the pledge not to abandon the patient—derive from the fundamental raison d'être of a physician, to do his or her best for the patient. Beneficence and the other physician requirements were traditionally thought of not merely as part of a business contract but as part of a trust—some would even say a covenant (Pellegrino and Thomasma 1988). Medicine is complex, decisions must be made quickly, and a patient cannot possibly know what his or her physician knows. Furthermore, illness itself may compromise clear thinking. Anxiety or depression not associated with the primary problem may lead to denial or other distortions of judgment. Thus the relationship was unequal because the patient, sick and vulnerable, had no choice but to accept it. The physician can be objective and subjective at the same time; he or she can understand a malady while empathizing with the bearer of that malady.

Two other central notions of the American cultural ethos are the individual-centered approach and compassion for fellow human beings in trouble. Although these can also be ascribed to traditional Western moral tenets, the particular emphasis of the young nation on solidarity driven by individuality is at the core of these beliefs. That the patient comes first is also an integral part of the World Health Organization's Declaration of Geneva (World Health Organization 1961) and of the preamble of the American Medical Association's Principles of Medical Ethics (American Medical Association Council on Ethical and Judicial Affairs 1998) and has also been the cornerstone of the doctor-patient relationship throughout the ages (American Psychiatric Association 1998; Lain-Entralgo 1968). Nevertheless, it is now evident that these and other aspects of traditional American medical ethics are under increasing strain because of the various ways and mechanisms introduced into the practice of medicine and psychiatry by managed care philosophies and policies.

Another important feature of American culture—that of free enterprise fed by competitiveness and guided by the concept of acquisition of wealth as an individual right, according to the Protestant version of profits and the work ethic—has presided over the evolution of the United States health care system. That individual initiatives should reflect and indeed be promoted with a minimum of government interference is a sacred mandate of American life. The health care system cannot be an exception, and, therefore, notable among its main features are its largely private structure, enhanced by the lowest taxes in the industrialized world, and free market–based operations. The diverse and complex set of treatment modalities that emerged as a result created an unprecedented wealth for health care–providing institutions and practitioners between the 1940s and the 1960s. This growth, however, did collide with the need for a rational organization and orderly delivery and cost of services. A militant pluralism prevented an effective coordination of the system's financial structure. A growing heterogeneity of values among the citizens led to what may be, from an ethical perspective, a significant omission: the United States, unlike almost all other industrialized countries, has never determined that health care is an individual right. Only in the last few years has the government made clear its intention to create a patient bill of rights and to advocate principles that should be not only wholly understood but implicit in every approach to health care policy making.

There are more factors that help one to understand the United States health care system as a patchwork of different modalities with not a few paradoxical implications. For example, although the United States devotes a greater percentage of its gross national product to health care than does any other industrialized country, less than half of those health care expenditures are government based (compared with an average of 76% in the rest of the industrial world) and there are large numbers of uninsured people (more than 40 million, and 17% of nonelderly individuals as of 1990) (Iglehart 1992). Furthermore, health care costs began to rise in the late 1960s and increased tremendously over the next two and a half decades. In 1960, health care costs were 4.6% of the gross national product, by 1970 they were 7.0%, and they had reached 13.9% by 1994. Some factors mentioned as causes for this tremendous increase in costs were the aging of the population, greater use of technology, and an unprecedented growth in the number of lawsuits. Increasingly, however, many believed that the fundamental reason for the continuing escalation of health care costs was the structure of the payment system— that is, health care was largely paid for by third parties or insurance companies and therefore patients and their physicians were shielded from considerations of the cost of care (Morrein 1995; Stoline 1998). Again, the ethical corollary of these developments is unmistakable.

The development and organization of health care mirrored the conflicting cultural values of a society guided by compassion and solidarity but also by individualism and competitiveness, a society that believed in the value of hard work but also in the hedonistic complacencies of wealth, a society profoundly religious but also multidimensionally sensuous, a society whose historical advancement was based on the exploration of endlessly open frontiers but whose citizens feverishly defended their right to privacy (Moore 1978). American society gave the medical profession free rein in the administration of fees and care costs, while maintaining an unquestioning faith in the moral precepts of medical practice. Gradually, however, the same society also gave free rein to health care entrepreneurs (many of them nurtured in the growing corporate mentality) as they entered the market and started taking price and cost controls away from the individual practitioner. Hospital-based care, promoted by an insatiable health insurance industry, began to be the norm for the middle and working classes. To complicate matters, health insurance policies between the 1960s and 1980s paid as any kind of insurance does—that is, retrospectively, after medical services have been rendered; for many years, those policies paid whatever was billed by physicians and hospitals. Employer-paid health insurance was never government mandated but was mostly the result of bargaining between unions and management. The stage was then set for the existence of disparate, sometimes overlapping systems covering different groups with different criteria, different organization of care, and different payment methods—private insurance, Medicare, Medicaid, public city hospitals, self-pay, military coverage, coverage for veterans, the Indian Health Service, and many more. Self-employed people were also buying insurance from a great variety of insurance carriers.

There have been several attempts, particularly in the last few decades, to create a government-paid national health insurance system. All of these attempts, however, were defeated by either an indecisive public (lured by sometimes unrealistic promises by the private sector's costly advertising campaigns), weak politicians returning favors to corporate donors, or the constant invocation of cultural and moral beliefs in the fairness of the American system, the honesty of government agencies and private corporations, the moral integrity of individual practitioners, freedom of enterprise, cultivation of creative solutions in a mosaic of pluralistic options, and an unabated belief in a mythic and eternal spring of wealth. As recently as 1994, the government, under pressure from its foes, pulled out of its attempts at health care reform. However, government plans targeting particular groups have been in effect for several decades: Medicare for the elderly, Medicaid for the poor, and coverage for the military and through other federal agencies, and the Veterans Health Administration. These efforts were aimed at counteracting the private insurance model of essentially cost-plus coverage for the same populations.

How did psychiatric patients and mental health care costs fare in the middle of this evolution? Not surprisingly, they differed—sometimes significantly—from those in mainstream practices. Based almost entirely in psychiatric hospitals, psychiatric practice was extremely well organized institutionally, and for more than 100 years its practitioners have been militant in their demands for humanistic and humane care. That this was a setting for the teaching of basic ethical principles was obvious, and the reception of ideas such as the "moral treatment" of nineteenth-century Europe was more than favorable (Micale and Porter 1994). Since early in the history of the country, mentally ill patients were largely marginal groups of society, vilified by stigma, hidden out of guilt or shame, or protected through society's paternalism. The confinement of the psychiatric practice meant there was only minimal impact on the actual attitudes in American society toward persons with mental illness. The youthful optimism of the new nation almost forced it to hide what in many cases was either unexplainable or considered the result of evil forces, sinfulness, or other unmanageable factors. Silence, isolation, selective deafness, or plain ignorance on the part of a populace very busy in building its own sources of wealth were convenient cover-up mechanisms or sophisticated rationalizations. The cultural belief in personal privacy was here an extraordinarily important factor.

After World War II, the destigmatization of at least minor psychological problems and the concomitant growth of office practice (aided by insurance payments) made private care the major component of psychiatric care. Thus began the reconvergence of psychiatry with the rest of medicine. Psychiatry and medicine were then subject to a payment system guided by the private free market, a supposedly fair and apparently solid organization that lacked, however, the necessary cost discipline of a true free market.

The Era of Managed Care

The foregoing discussion has amply demonstrated that for many decades the traditional American medical codes and practices were based on a patient-centered beneficence and a practitioner-generated paternalism. These took place in the midst of a culture based on autonomy as manifested in free-market precepts and an individualistic creed. Interestingly enough, these two currents evolved during the 1960s into increasing power for patients. The physician authority—also based on the same principles of free enterprise, individualism, and autonomy—gradually fostered patient autonomy, with the support of legal and bioethical principles. An example of these conflicting developments was the change in commitment and in voluntary treatment laws that resulted in precedent-setting court decisions protecting the patient's integrity as well as in a nascent patient bill of rights (Miller 1987).

The era of patient autonomy, fueled by all the historical, social, institutional, economic, and ethical changes described previously, set the stage for managed care. Patient autonomy was the clarion call in the campaign to weaken what was considered the excessive power of physicians. Examples of this movement were the promotion of contract models of medical care in the 1970s, and the unstoppable growth of third-party health insurance payers, paralleled by the growth of Medicare and Medicaid as government-initiated counteractions. Other efforts such as institution of deductibles, copayments, or prior approval for tests and hospitalizations did not slow the spiraling of health care costs. The revolt of the payers mounted up to a demand that they have ultimate control. Because this was practically impossible, the stage was set for another force to erupt into the scene: managed care organizations, "a wide range of review and service delivery systems designed to control health care costs by controlling the utilization of health care resources" (Stoline 1998, pp. 12–13). This followed the failure of the Clinton administration's attempt at health care reform, paradoxically having almost identical goals, namely containing costs, covering more individual lives, achieving parity and universality of care coverage, and promoting efficiency and even higher levels of excellence in the middle of an evident economic bonanza.

The managed care philosophy is simple in its basic points. The goal is to promote efficiency and quality in patient care while reducing costs. It involves a capitation approach to health care budgets for individuals, employees, corporations, and a variety of other groups. Managed care creates incentives for practitioners and patients, fosters competition, claims to be patient-centered and essentially driven by patient preferences and satisfaction, and a declared willingness to flexibility and relatively quick change. It is based on quantitative, survey-based approaches, use of forms and clinical protocols based on a continuously improving technology. It is also based on the gathering of the largest possible number of practitioners in different fields and geographic locations. There is an emphasis on good-quality care, but also on preventive measures, patient and public education, and the use of primary care practitioners either as gatekeepers or as primary providers.

The physician's work is influenced by different means of control of clinical decisions and incentives. Reimbursement for a restricted range of drugs, the necessity of second opinions for expensive tests or procedures, and utilization review are some of these approaches (Morrein 1995). Clinical protocols can be modified according to a variety of criteria (e.g., costs, patient response, or new research findings). Managed care is basically a market-based approach to health care and, as such, includes a corporate mentality with profits for the stockholders as its main essential goal.

Another by-product of the managed care era is the creation of a new jargon. Physicians were initially called "care providers" and are now called "care managers." Primary care practitioners are called *gatekeepers*. The patient is the "client" or "customer," and groups of patients and the public at large are one of several groups of "stakeholders." Capitation-based budgets are there to be spent at the minimum and, in a dramatic twist of word meaning, an intervention or "encounter" with the "customer" is designated a "loss."

Reaction of the professional community.   If breaking the physician's authority and influence was one of the objectives of managed care, it can be said that such a goal has been accomplished with various levels of success. Depicted initially as villains, physicians in many cases have been moved to salaried positions and, what is worst in the opinion of managed care critics, have seen their professional autonomy and decision-making capabilities drastically reduced, subjected as they now are to so-called evidence-based medicine, disease management guidelines, and similar restrictions. Professional organizations such as the American Medical Association and the American Psychiatric Association have reacted strongly to this trend. In fact, the American Psychiatric Association has established a hotline for educating practitioners about the vagaries of managed care and for gathering complaints of sound ethical impact. Thus the ethical implications and challenges posed to the psychiatric practice by managed care have been documented primarily with regard to quality of care—that is, to whether managed care has met the real expectations of the consumer (American Psychiatric Association Committee on Managed Care 1992).

Individual practitioners and groups of practitioners have also reacted against the abuses of managed care. They invoke moral principles, particularly the assault against individual autonomy (both of the patient and the practitioner), and the subsequent severe harming of human dignity, the drama of human suffering, and the callousness of rigid policies enforced by ill-informed bureaucrats. Alternative proposals to counteract managed care have gone from Canadian-style single-payer systems and medical savings accounts, to market-based approaches to health care (e.g., physician service organizations, behavioral group practices, independent practice associations, management service organizations, physician hospital organizations, physician service networks, and physician-owned insurance companies) (Schreter 1998). All of them are designed to give back control of clinical decision-making to the physician by eliminating the managed care intermediary and external watchdogs. Needless to say, strong community ties are also advised as yet another strategy.

Ethical challenges and battles.   Managed care is a challenge to the psychiatric profession that resulted fundamentally from the increasing inability of medicine to set its own ethics and conditions of work at a doable and universally acceptable level. The challenge extends to the ethical arena at several levels:

+ *Double agentry.* The practitioner finds himself or herself serving two masters: the patient and the managed care organization. In traditional medical ethics, the physician's loyalty is undivided: the patient is first priority. Whereas this basic allegiance demands the use of every means possible to help the patient, managed care organization rules and policies encourage taking the least costly approaches to save money that could eventually result in greater income and incentives. The managed care organization is a business whose stockholders certainly expect profits (Angell 1987; Levinsky 1984). Paradoxically, recent experiences show that profits are not being made, which thus increases the pressure to augment premium policy costs.

♦ *Fidelity*. Fidelity entails loyalty to the profession's basic ethical principles symbolized by the patient in need. The dichotomy of the "two masters" may lead to an endless series of rationalizations aimed at justifying the psychiatrist's role in particular circumstances for a particular case. The doctor-patient relationship suffers, because patients cannot be trusting in situations in which their physicians are not entirely on their side (Crawshaw et al. 1995). Probably the most satisfactory way to resolve the dilemmas of fidelity is to move the system toward a focus on quality of care as a competitive edge for managed care organizations rather than purely cost; the history of American business would indicate that this is likely.

♦ *Confidentiality*. Confidentiality as a supreme ethical principle for any medical practitioner is compromised by the demands of the market reflected in changes by consumers, variations in policies, documentation of interventions, administrative supervision, billing and collections, and so on. This is made even more complicated by the expectation of thorough information subjected to the dictates of practice guidelines. Omissions are strongly punished in financial terms or in paying policies, and details are expected in ways that betray the essentials of confidentiality (Hall and Berenson 1998). Furthermore, nonmedical people at administrative or bureaucratic levels feel entitled to know what is going on.

♦ *Informed consent*. A clear example of the ethical constraints imposed by managed care are the limitations of coverage stipulated by insurance policies or other requirements documented in the form known as the informed consent. Forced by the group insurance approach, individual employees, for instance, must abdicate a number of areas of coverage in the name of cost and efficiency. One way of disguising this disadvantageous situation is to place an emphasis on personal autonomy, personal choice, and freedom of choice for the patient regarding procedures that are described as dangerous (Kassirer 1998). It is well known, for example, that in many states of the Union, electroconvulsive therapy is simply prohib-

ited, thus denying both individual freedom of choice and clinical experience and scientific proof.

◆ *Honesty.* There is no question that honesty can be imperiled by the ethically narrow set of rules imposed by managed care. "Gaming the system"
sometimes becomes a way for both the patient and the psychiatrist to ensure coverage that is not specifically stated in the policies. False or exag-
gerated claims of care are reported in order to alleviate lesser conditions or
make illegal use of treatment resources. The erosion of other ethical principles appears to be a clear risk, because competence and compassion dic-
tate new duties for doctors: disclosure of their financial incentives to their
patients, advocacy with their managed care company, and careful review
of any agreements they might make with managed care organizations
(Morrein 1995).

◆ *Vulnerability.* Psychiatric practice is particularly vulnerable to managed
care policies. A clear example is psychotherapy, which is already done by
other mental health professionals, to the detriment of the psychiatrist's
identity, technical skills, training, and availability. This situation, based exclusively on the lesser costs of services provided by nonpsychiatric mental
health professionals, also creates the potential for a lowering of the various
quality-of-care standards that managed care claims to protect. Professional self-esteem is also undermined, and the desirable joint work of different professionals becomes more a source of dissension, divisiveness,
and distractive competition.

Conclusions

The same culture that led to present-day managed care practices may be the
source of much-needed corrections. It is not a matter of demonizing managed
care on the basis of hostility and spitefulness. Rescuing basic or essential managed care precepts is as important a factor in the development of professional
practice as it is in the field of ethics. The balanced view of dual agentry, confidentiality, fidelity, honesty, and vulnerability is in itself an ethical imperative.
Sabin (1996) proposed four principles to supplement the psychiatric code of
ethics for use by psychiatrists practicing in managed care situations. They address the psychiatrist's role as a faithful doctor to his or her patients and as a
"steward of society's resources"; the use of least-costly treatments unless
there is "substantial evidence" for a superior outcome with costlier interventions; justice in the health care system; and use of "explicit standards" to
withhold beneficial interventions.

The autonomy of the profession of psychiatry is a conflicting and conflicted area and it must be protected as much as the patient's well-being. In recent months, increasing protests by the public toward managed care's selfish practices have even found their way into the courts, strengthening the position of those who say that a degree of regulation in the name of fairness and ethics is mandatory and almost unavoidable. The future of psychiatry—is it a profession or a corporation?—is also at stake, with many if not all practitioners of course sticking to the professional identity based on unmovable, essential ethical principles. A reformulation of sacred documents about ethical standards of the profession—from the Hippocratic Oath to the 1996 Declaration of Madrid (see the Appendix to this book)—in more precise and contemporary terms is a critical step. To sum up, the duty of the psychiatrist to inform and advise, maintain confidentiality, be in partnership with the patient, choose the right therapeutic modality, and provide the best available care consistent with accepted scientific knowledge and ethical principles will only reinforce his or her individual sense of responsibility and the discharge of his or her duties under the highest moral standards. A vigilant profession may in the end be the best guarantee for the people it serves. Thus cultural principles and ethical norms would have converged for the genuine healing of society as a whole.

References

Ackerknecht E: A Short History of Psychiatry. New York, Hafner, 1968

Alarcon RD: Cultural and psychiatric diagnosis: impact on DSM-IV and ICD-10. Psychiatr Clin North Am 18:449–465, 1995

American Medical Association Council on Ethical and Judicial Affairs: Code of Medical Ethics. Chicago, IL, American Medical Association, 1998

American Psychiatric Association: Diagnostic and Statistical Manual of Mental Disorders, 3rd Edition. Washington, DC, American Psychiatric Association, 1980

American Psychiatric Association: Diagnostic and Statistical Manual of Mental Disorders, 3rd Edition, Revised. Washington, DC, American Psychiatric Association, 1987

American Psychiatric Association: Diagnostic and Statistical Manual of Mental Disorders, 4th Edition. Washington, DC, American Psychiatric Association, 1994

American Psychiatric Association: The Principles of Medical Ethics, With Annotations Especially Applicable to Psychiatry. Washington, DC, American Psychiatric Press, 1998

American Psychiatric Association Committee on Managed Care: Utilization Management: A Handbook for Psychiatrists. Washington, DC, American Psychiatric Association, 1992

Angell M: Medicine: the endangered patient-centered ethic. Hastings Cent Rep 17 (suppl):12–13, 1987

Billington R: Westward Expansion. New York, New York University Press, 1949

Blain B, Barton D: The History of American Psychiatry: A Teaching and Research Guide. Washington, DC, American Psychiatric Association, 1979

Carter RT: The Influence of Race and Racial Identity in Psychotherapy: Toward a Racially Inclusive Model. New York, Wiley, 1995

Clark JJ: On the unity and diversity of cultures. American Anthropologist 72:545–554, 1970

Crawshaw R, Rogers DE, Pellegrino ED, et al: Patient-physician covenant. JAMA 273:1553, 1995

Hall MA, Berenson RA: Ethical practice in managed care: a dose of realism. Ann Intern Med 128:395–402, 1998

Iglehart JK: The American health care system: introduction. N Engl J Med 326:962–967, 1992

Kassirer JP: Managed care—should we adopt a new ethic? N Engl J Med 339:397–398, 1998

Lain-Entralgo P: Doctor-Patient Relationship. New York, Columbia University Press, 1968

Levinsky NG: The doctor's master. N Engl J Med 311:1573–1575, 1984

Maybury-Lewis D: Millennium, Tribal Wisdom and the Modern World. New York, WW Norton, 1992

Micale MS, Porter R (eds): Discovering the History of Psychiatry. New York, Oxford University Press, 1994

Miller RD: Involuntary Commitment of the Mentally Ill in the Post-reform Era. Springfield, IL, Charles C Thomas, 1987

Moore RA: Ethics in the practice of psychiatry—origins, functions, models, and enforcement. Am J Psychiatry 135:157–163, 1978

Morrein EH: Balancing Act: The New Ethics of Medicine's New Economics. Georgetown University Press, Washington, DC, 1995

Parrington VL: Main Currents in American Thought. New York, Atheneum, 1930

Pellegrino EP, Thomasma DC: For the Patient's Good: The Restoration of Beneficence in Health Care. New York, Oxford University Press, 1988

Pessen E: The egalitarian myth and the American social reality: wealth, mobility and equality in the "era of the common man." American History Review 76:989–1034, 1971

Potter D: History and American Society. New York, Columbia University Press, 1973

Sabin JE: Is managed care ethical care? in Controversies in Managed Mental Health Care. Edited by Lazarus A. Washington, DC, American Psychiatric Press, 1996, pp 115–126

Schor JB: The Overspent American. New York, Basic Books, 1998

Schreter RK: Uncertain market opens the door for new strategies in promoting wellness. Eco Facts 2:3–6, 1998

Stoline AM: The emergence of organized systems of care, in New Roles for Psychiatrists in Organized Systems of Care. Edited by Lazarus JA, Sharfstein SS. Washington, DC, American Psychiatric Press, 1998, pp 3–22

Torrey EF, Erdman K, Wolfe S, et al: Care of the Seriously Mentally Ill: A Rating of State Programs, 3rd Edition. Washington, DC, Public Citizen Health Research Group and National Alliance for the Mentally Ill, 1990

Trinterud LJ: The Forming of an American Tradition: A Re-examination of Colonial Presbyterianism. Philadelphia, PA, University of Pennsylvania Press, 1949

Walters RG: American Reformers, 1815–1860. New York, New York University Press, 1978

Weber M: The Protestant Ethic and the Spirit of Capitalism. New York, Basic Books, 1930

Wilson M: DSM-III and the transformation of American psychiatry: a history. Am J Psychiatry 150:399–410, 1993

Wittels F: The contribution of Benjamin Rush to psychiatry. Bull Hist Med 20:157–166, 1946

World Health Organization: Declaration of Geneva. Geneva, World Health Organization, 1961

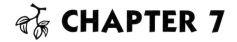 **CHAPTER 7**

Ethics in Sub-Saharan Africa

Prof. Michael O. Olatawura

Because *ethics* refers to a system of morals or rules of behavior, it is educative to examine the implications of this definition for medical practice, particularly psychiatric practice in different cultures. In terms of ethics, there are certain minimum standards expected of every doctor. The following 14 duties are the requirements of any doctor registered with the General Medical Council of the United Kingdom (1997):

1. Doctors must make the care of their patients their first concern.
2. They must treat every patient politely and considerately.
3. They must respect patients' dignity and privacy.
4. They must listen to patients and respect their views.
5. They must give patients information in a way they can understand.
6. They must respect the rights of patients to be fully involved in decisions about their care.
7. They must keep their professional knowledge and skills up to date.
8. They must recognize the limits of their professional competence.
9. They must be honest and trustworthy.
10. They must respect and protect confidential information.
11. They must make sure that their personal beliefs do not prejudice their patients' care.
12. They must act quickly to protect patients from risk if they have good reason to believe that they or their colleagues may not be fit to practice.

13. They must avoid abusing their positions as doctors.
14. They must work with their colleagues in the ways that best serve patients' interests.

To understand the implications of some of these ethical requirements for psychiatric practice in West Africa, one must know something about African culture. Culture is an abstraction that encompasses the total way of life of a society. "It is a precipitate of the group's history and expresses its adaptation to the physical environment. It is characterized by a psychological reality which refers to the shared patterns of belief, feeling and knowledge, i.e., the basic values, axioms and assumptions that members of the group carry in their mind as guides for conduct and the definition of reality (Benedict 1934, Hallowell 1955, and Snow 1959)" (cited by Leighton and Murphy 1965, p. 15).

History of Sub-Saharan African Culture

The constituent tribes of each of the sub-Saharan African countries are many and varied within themselves; ethnic delineation can be very sharp. In Nigeria, which has a population of about 100 million, there are well over 300 dialects spoken; these dialects can be so distinct that people in geographically close ethnic groups that make up a tribe may not understand each other's language. These points highlight the fact that there must be differences in ways of life among the people of sub-Saharan Africa, namely French-, English-, Portuguese-, and Spanish-speaking people. Like everywhere else, life in the region was simple at first, the main preoccupations of the population being to survive the vicissitudes of nature and to deal with territorial conflicts. In Africa in general, ways of life were heavily influenced by great reverence for the spirit world, populated by departed souls of ancestors. Animism guided Africans' thoughts, wishes, aspirations, and fears. Social order in primitive societies was guided and guaranteed by taboos and totems (i.e., objects of superstitious respect).

Because initially nothing was written, the customs and traditions—the culture—of each tribe were passed on orally. Because the elders were the custodians of these customs and traditions, they were highly venerated. To a large degree, this has remained true of all African societies, the impact of western education and civilization notwithstanding. This explains the respect that Africans have for the opinions of their fathers, mothers, uncles, aunts, and elders in general. When the opinion is that of a grandparent, it is virtually inviolable; it has the force of a decree.

Impact of Culture on Perception of Health and Disease

Africans believe that to maintain good health, both physical and mental, they must maintain contact with their ancestors, the spirit world, through activities such as propitiation and other rituals at prescribed periods throughout the year. Thus to ward off epidemics that decimate childhood populations; failed harvests (resulting in famine); natural catastrophes such as floods and earthquakes; premature death; mental illness; infertility; and so on, taboos are applied and rituals and festivals are carried out. When these approaches are taken, the society enjoys peace and harmony. Given that the family is the smallest unit of every society, the African family plays a major part in the following of cultural dictates. As previously mentioned, elderly persons are highly venerated. Men have their prescribed role, as do elderly women in the family. Younger members of traditional African families cannot make certain decisions, particularly in the area of health care, without referring to authority figures in the family. In the case of sickness, it may be the grandfather or grandmother who is the authority figure. A wife cannot give consent for any treatment, whether scientific or traditional, without the knowledge of her husband, even in an emergency.

The implications that African culture has for recognition of ill health, diagnosis, and management must be made clear to some extent. There is another dimension, namely that the colleagues of African psychiatrists are not only their surgical and internist colleagues but also traditional and faith healers. In discussing the impact of culture on ethics and psychiatry, one must reconsider the 14 duties of a doctor as articulated by the General Medical Council of the United Kingdom. Care of the patient in sub-Saharan Africa is the concern not only of the psychiatrist but of the family as well as traditional and faith healers. In many instances, the latter two have a higher profile than does the psychiatrist. Maintaining the patient's privacy and dignity can be difficult because the "sanctity" of the psychiatrist's hospital ward cannot be guaranteed, especially when African governments and their citizenry require that conventional and alternative medical practitioners collaborate and cooperate.

Of course, quite often the psychiatrist has the usual full liberty, practicing in the privacy of his or her office. Even then, however, the patient's views are more often than not the views of the elders in the family. African patients tend to understand the information given to them by traditional and faith healers because they share the same view of illness and disease and what should be done to remove or lessen suffering. This view is held even by African patients with M.D. or Ph.D. degrees. Thus the patient is only partially involved in decisions about his or her care. An African psychiatrist's beliefs may clash with his or her ethical position. The psychiatrist may be conflicted when he or she suspects that the traditional and faith-healing practices, embraced by the family of the patient, may not be in the patient's best interest. At present, African psychiatrists spend much time on health education to persuade their compatriots that although supernatural forces could be at play, diseases and infections should be excluded before patients are treated with traditional and faith healing. Adhering to the "pure" ethics of conventional medicine is not an enviable task for African psychiatrists.

Selected Issues

Admission of a severely psychotic patient is usually at the insistence of the patient's family. The family usually makes the decision about where to seek help, whether at a psychiatric facility or at a traditional healer's.

As indicated earlier, the attribution of mental illness to factors such as witchcraft or breaking of taboos creates ethical problems for the psychiatrist, who is obliged to provide the most up-to-date information to African patients and their relatives. Although most African psychiatrists do not dismiss entirely some of the traditional beliefs regarding mental illness, they hold the conventional position with regard to etiology and treatment, in particular, when relatives and patients ask for information and when explanations are necessary for drug compliance and rehabilitation. There is really no conflict here. Moreover, the African psychiatrist believes that the traditional explanations of the origin of psychiatric illness accepted both by the patient and his or her relatives and by the traditional healer permit greater psychotherapeutic achievements by the traditional healer. Thus the psychiatrist emphasizes the importance of medication compliance while not discouraging the use of the traditional healer.

Homosexuality is by and large seen as a disorder in sub-Saharan Africa. African gays and lesbians may now get some relief from their psychological "symptoms" because Western media are getting the message across to Africans that homosexuality is neither a disorder nor a sin.

As in the rest of the world, substance use disorders are a big problem. The problem has increased and become more complex with the arrival of hard drugs. Also, the health delivery program in Africa is unable to cope with the basic health needs, much less substance-use disorders, of its massive population.

Declaration of Madrid and Ethical Psychiatric Practice

The first point in the Declaration of Madrid (see the Appendix to this book) highlights the fact that the best treatment, including rehabilitation of mentally ill patients, should be the watchword of every psychiatrist.

Because of very poor financial allocation to health care in general and mental health care in particular by governments in sub-Saharan Africa, as in many other parts of the developing world, efforts of psychiatrists are severely curtailed. All that is possible at the moment in this region is the shortening of episodes of psychiatric illness by means of physical treatment, namely administration of psychotropic drugs and electroconvulsive therapy.

For decades, poor allocation of funds to health institutions and universities has hampered research and hindered the keeping abreast, through reading of journals, of the latest developments in psychiatry.

The much hallowed therapist-patient relationship is undermined in sub-Saharan Africa by the usual culturally dictated reserve of the African patient, sometimes amounting to abdication of freedom to make informed decisions. Married female patients must obtain permission from their husbands to follow their doctors' advice. The form of treatment is often a matter to be decided by the elders in the patient's family. The extended family of the African patient, rather than the patient himself or herself, often occupies center stage in these situations.

Even when the patient is deemed capable of exercising proper judgment, the African psychiatrist more often than not will make headway by consulting the family. In situations of doubtful testamentary capacity, due process of the law is invoked by the psychiatrist. Treatment that the African psychiatrist thinks is not in the best interest of the patient cannot always be successfully argued against by the psychiatrist. The family of the patient is not prevented by law from signing for the discharge of the patient against medical advice. For example, relatives may opt for faith healing or traditional healing in situations in which the patient requires antibiotics and other physical resuscitative measures.

When asked to assess a patient, the African psychiatrist makes no ethical compromises in terms of withholding information given to him or her in confidence by the patient. The rights and autonomy of psychiatric patients as research subjects are well protected by institutional ethical committee safeguards. Currently, issues such as euthanasia, torture, the death penalty, selection of sex, and organ transplantation are virtually nonissues for psychiatrists in sub-Saharan Africa.

References

Benedict R: Patterns of Culture. Boston, Houghton Mifflin, 1934

General Medical Council: Annual Review. London, UK, General Medical Council, 1997

Hallowell AJ: Culture and Experience. Philadelphia, PA, University of Pennsylvania Press, 1955

Leighton AH, Murphy JM: Approaches to Cross-Cultural Psychiatry. Ithaca, NY, Cornell University Press, 1965

Snow CP: The Two Cultures and the Scientific Revolution. New York, Cambridge University Press, 1959

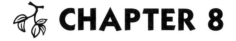 CHAPTER 8

The Indian Experience

Prof. R. Srinivasa Murthy

During the last three decades, there has been a major change in the practice of psychiatry all over the world. In the Western world, the manner of provision of care to persons with mental illness is being rethought; there has been a shift from institutional care to community care and there is growing awareness of the rights of mentally ill individuals. In the developing countries of Asia and Africa, there are beginnings of organizations for universal coverage of mental health care (Srinivasa Murthy 1996). In these initiatives, both the strengths of traditional societies and advances in mental health knowledge have been used.

These two developments have brought into focus the contrasts between universal and local aspects of psychiatry (Sullivan 1989). The importance of traditional societies, in terms of how behavior of and care for people with mental disorders are interpreted, has received attention, as has the expansion of mental health programs. As a result, there are universal guidelines with local variations.

There is evidence that interest among psychiatrists in the ethical foundations of their work has escalated in the past two to three decades. This interest may be greater than in any other period of the history of psychiatry. Several factors have contributed to this new interest: the medical consumer movement, the civil liberties movement, changes in treatment settings, debates about informed consent, political use of psychiatry, the changing conception of confidentiality because of insurance policies, and changes in law, sociology, psychology, theology, and philosophy (Bloch and Chodoff 1991).

In this chapter, I focus on five aspects: the Indian approach to medical ethics, Indian initiatives in developing medical ethical guidelines, Indian psychiatrists' approach to psychiatric ethics, emerging mental health programs in India, and the implications of these developments for the international psychiatric ethics movement.

Wig (1999) considered in detail some of the important features of Indian philosophy as they relate to mental health. The major ways in which Indian philosophy differs from Western philosophical traditions are described here:

♦ The chief mark of Indian philosophy is its concentration on the spiritual. Both in life and in philosophy, the spiritual motive is predominant. Neither humanity nor the universe is looked on as physical in essence, and material welfare is never recognized as the only goal of human life.

♦ In India, philosophy and religion are intimately related. Philosophy is never considered merely an intellectual exercise. In every Indian system, truth is sought not in a quest for academic knowledge but out of a desire to learn the truth, which shall make us free.

♦ Indian philosophy is characterized by an introspective approach to reality. In pursuit of truth, Indian philosophy has been strongly dominated by concern with the inner life and the human self rather than the external world of physical nature.

♦ Indian philosophy is essentially idealistic. The tendency of Indian philosophy, especially Hinduism, has been toward monistic idealism. In almost all schools of Indian philosophy, reality is believed to be ultimately one and spiritual.

♦ Indian philosophy makes unquestioned and extensive use of reason, but intuition is accepted as the major method through which the ultimate can be known. Reason and intellectual knowledge are not enough. Reason is not useless or fallacious, but it is insufficient. To know reality, one must have actual experience of it. One does not merely know the truth in Indian philosophy; one must realize it and live it.

♦ Indian philosophy is dominated by synthetic tradition, which is essential to the spirit and method of Indian philosophy. According to Indian tradition, true religion comprehends all religions; hence the famous Sanskrit saying, "God is one, but men call him by many names."

Ethical aspects of Hinduism were considered by Reddy (1998) and Weiss (1994). Ethics in Hinduism are derived from certain spiritual concepts and form the foundation of the spiritual life. Hindu ethics differ both from modern scientific ethics, which are largely influenced by biology (i.e., whatever is conducive to continuous survival of a particular individual or species is considered good for it), and from utilitarian ethics, which are chiefly concerned with society. Hindu ethics are mainly subjective or personal. The purpose of them is to eliminate mental impurities such as greed, egotism, cruelty, and ruthlessness. Ethical disciplines are prescribed according to the stage and state of each person.

In Hinduism, more emphasis is placed on personal or subjective ethics than on social ethics, for the following reasons: 1) If individuals are virtuous, social welfare will follow as a matter of course. 2) The general moral tone in Hinduism is that everyone is expected to carry out his or her appropriate duties, which include rendering help to less fortunate fellow human beings. Spiritual help is of more enduring value than material help. Those with spiritual knowledge who apply subjective or personal ethics can easily bear physical pain and privations, and they do so with calmness and patience. 3) Lastly, the Hindu philosophers believe that the sum total of physical happiness and suffering remains constant.

The chief components of subjective ethics are austerity, self-control, renunciation, nonattachment, and concentration. Austerity helps an individual to curb impulses for inordinate enjoyment of physical comforts and engage in intense thinking before creative work, making an individual indifferent about his or her personal comforts or discomforts. Self-control means guiding one's senses, choosing the right objects by discrimination, being determined, and developing dispassion.

Objective ethics are a means to an end. The purpose is to help members of society rid themselves of self-centeredness. Among the social virtues, hospitality, courtesy, and duties to the family and community are stressed. In Hinduism, leading an ethical life means living simply; not being greedy; being charitable, compassionate, gentle, and pious; acting in consideration of the welfare of others; providing succor to distressed persons; being of service to all; and bearing no ill will toward others (Reddy 1998).

Ethical Guidelines for Biomedical Research

Ethical considerations of medical research have been the subject of concern among Indian medical professionals. In 1980, the Indian Council of Medical Research brought out a document entitled "Policy Statement on Ethical Considerations Involved in Research on Human Subjects." This was the guiding document until recently.

In 1996, the Indian Council of Medical Research (1997) created a central ethical committee to review the 1980 guidelines and to focus on four major areas: human genetics research, transplantation research, clinical evaluation of drugs, and epidemiological research. The committee reviewed the ethical, legal, social, and other issues of research involving or affecting human subjects, and formulated general and specific principles for research.

The general principles identified as central are essentiality; voluntariness, informed consent, and community agreement; nonexploitation; privacy and confidentiality; risk minimization; professional competence; accountability and transparency; maximization of public interest and of distributive justice; institutional arrangements; availability of information in the public domain; totality of responsibility; and compliance.

Psychiatric Initiatives

The Indian Lunacy Act (Government of India 1912) was replaced by the Mental Health Act (Government of India 1987). Chapter 8 of the Mental Health Act covers the protection of rights of mentally ill persons:

1. No mentally ill person shall be subjected during treatment to any indignity (whether physical or mental) or cruelty.
2. No mentally ill person under treatment shall be used for purposes of research unless:

   i. such research is of direct benefit to him for purposes of diagnosis or treatment; or
   ii. such person, being a voluntary patient, has given his consent in writing or where such person (whether or not a voluntary patient) is incompetent, by reason of minority or otherwise, to give valid consent, the guardian or other person competent to give consent on his behalf, has given his consent in writing, for such research and

3. Subject to any rules made on this behalf under Section 94 for the purpose of preventing vexatious or defamatory communications or communications prejudicial to the treatment of mentally ill persons, no letters or other communications sent by or to mentally ill persons under treatment shall be intercepted, detained or destroyed. (Government of India 1987)

Indian Psychiatric
Society Ethical Guidelines

The Indian Psychiatric Society adopted the following ethical guidelines for psychiatrists in 1989:

Preamble

Ethics has been an essential part of the healing art. Ethical guidelines have been prepared by international and national organizations for different groups of practitioners. Each country has its own social, economic, and psychological compulsions, which might make it difficult to translate and practice ethical codes of other countries. Hence this body proposes the following ethical guidelines for members of the psychiatric profession in this country. These principles are intended to aid psychiatrists individually and collectively in maintaining a high level of ethical conduct. They are not laws but standards by which psychiatrists may determine the propriety of their conduct and relationships with patients, with members of allied professions, and with the public.

Principles

1. *Responsibility:* As a practitioner, the psychiatrist must know that he bears a heavy social responsibility because he not only deals with disturbed human behavior but also has to contend with intimacies of life. As a scientist he should serve the society through observation, investigation and experimentation with well planned and ethically carried out research.

2. *Competence:* The maintenance of high standards of professional competence is the responsibility of all psychiatrists in the interest of both the public and the profession. Psychiatrists are responsible for their own continuing education and should realize that theirs must be a lifetime learning.
   As a member of the profession, they will not violate ethical standards and when such violation comes to their notice, will take steps to correct it.

3. *Benevolence:* The interest of the patient and his health will stand paramount with them in their professional practices. Personal interest would find but a secondary place. Financial arrangements will never contravene professional standards. Psychiatrists will always safeguard the interests of the patient and the profession.

4. *Moral Standards:* They will, at all times, be responsive to the moral codes and expectations of the community they serve and will not let their behavior malign their profession in any way.

5. *Patient Welfare:* They will not treat a case that does not clearly fall within their competence. The patients they accept, they will treat with the best of their ability and with the highest regards for the patient's integrity and welfare of the communities in which they work.
   They will terminate the clinical or consulting relationship with the patient when it is reasonably clear to them that the patient is no longer benefiting from it.
   In case of referral, they will continue to feel responsible for the patient's welfare until the responsibility has been formally transferred.

6. *Confidentiality:* They will safeguard information about a patient that they have obtained in the course of their clinical work, teaching or research in order to safeguard the patient's interest and protect him from social stigma, discrimination and harm. They will treat this as a primary obligation and not reveal unto others any such information unless certain ethical conditions are met or when there is clear and imminent danger to an individual or society and then only to the appropriate authorities or concerned co-professionals. Confidentiality of the clinical records will be meticulously guarded and identity of the patients will not be revealed even in scientific communication. No data about a patient shall be ordinarily revealed to any agency without the consent of the patient or his family.

Recommendations

1. Every person who has attained the age of majority and who does not appear to have lost the ability of reason shall be assumed to be capable of giving consent.
   A patient should be taken up for medical evaluation and treatment with his consent. In case a patient, because of his mental illness, is unable to express valid consent, the psychiatrist may undertake to treat him with the consent of a person close to him who appears to be clearly interested in the welfare of the patient. The only exception to treating without consent would be in an emergency situation involving an immediate threat to the life or health of the patient or others. For purposes of research, the consent shall be obtained on the lines indicated above after satisfying the following:

a. The consent is entirely voluntary.

b. The patient can withdraw the consent at any stage.

c. Withdrawal of the consent shall not affect the interest of the patient.

2. The decision to hospitalize a patient will essentially rest on the consideration of his welfare and will also take into consideration legal administrative constraints as well as its social appropriateness.

3. Psychiatric treatment shall be initiated only on clinical considerations and shall be in accordance with scientific knowledge and professional ethics. The patient's welfare should be the primary factor determining the choice of the treatment modality. Should the specific modality not fall within the competence of a psychiatrist, he should refer the patient to a competent colleague. The termination of therapy also shall be determined on clinical consideration.

All treatment should be humane and never punitive. No psychiatrist shall refuse to treat in an emergency.

4. Gifts and gratifications from patients under treatment should not be accepted.

5. Any kind of sexual advance toward any patient is unethical.

6. In case of doubt or in situations where unconventional treatment procedures are contemplated, a second opinion must be obtained.

7. It is unethical to force contact upon patients during treatment.

8. Even when a patient has been referred by a legal or administrative authority or by the employer, the welfare of the patient will remain of paramount consideration. The patient should be informed of the purpose for which he is to be examined.

9. Basic human rights of the mentally retarded should not be subjected to unethical abridgement. Due ethical discretion should be exercised when advising such procedures as sterilization.

10. In this interest of the patient and the society, drug abusers who refuse to give consent may be treated with the consent of their relatives. Effort has to be made to motivate them for accepting treatment voluntarily. (Indian Psychiatric Society 1989)

These ethical codes must be implemented with sincerity. Central and regional ethical committees should be formed. These committees should consider complaints either from the public or from fellow professionals and then carefully investigate them.

Emerging Mental Health Programs

In 1947, for a population of more than 300 million, there were only 10,000 beds for psychiatric patients and only a handful of mental health professionals. In the past 50 years, the situation has changed significantly. Currently, there are about 5,000 mental health professionals and a wide variety of mental health initiatives in the country (Srinivasa Murthy 1996). The major developments relevant to ethics are the formation of the National Mental Health Program in 1982; the integration of mental health care into primary health care to provide essential mental health care to the entire population (this includes direct responsibility for mental health care by nonspecialists); the development of a wide variety of community care facilities; the use of volunteers in suicide prevention; emphasis on family care and responsibility of family members in care programs; a greater awareness of mental health issues in the media and among the general population; changes in mental health legislation (summarized earlier in the chapter), giving greater power to family members and professionals with regard to admission; and the Persons With Disabilities Act (Government of India 1996), in which mental illness is considered a disability.

All of these developments will challenge the traditional concepts of roles and responsibilities and require active dialogue and monitoring. This has yet to occur to an optimum extent.

Conclusions

India has a rich past and a very recent history of organized mental health care. The rich past includes the religious and philosophical wisdom and tradition, including a well-developed system of health (Ayurveda).

Many issues in modern medical practice were addressed in Hindu religious texts, codes of conduct, and Sanskrit treatises of Ayurveda. In the medical texts, responsibilities of the physician to society, patients, and colleagues were discussed and the professional nature of these interactions, distinctive social values, and political forces were recognized. Some current major concerns in Western medical ethics, such as the status of rational suicide, were considered in the context of Hindu traditions other than medicine (Weiss 1994).

Recent developments have occurred in modern health care in general and mental health care in particular. As a result, there are many levels of mental health care initiatives, with unclear boundaries, raising a number of ethical concerns. The dialogue has begun, and sensitivity and experiences of professionals, planners, patients, and other people must be part of this dialogue. The specific progress reviewed offers hope that the national-level initiatives will evolve against a background of international ethical guidelines.

References

Bloch S, Chodoff P: Psychiatric Ethics, 2nd Edition. New York, Oxford University Press, 1991

Government of India: Indian Lunacy Act. New Delhi, Government of India, 1912

Government of India: Mental Health Act. New Delhi, Government of India, 1987

Government of India: Persons With Disabilities Act. New Delhi, Government of India, 1996

Indian Council of Medical Research: Policy Statement on Ethical Considerations Involved in Research on Human Subjects. New Delhi, Indian Council of Medical Research, 1980

Indian Council of Medical Research: Consultative Document on Ethical Guidelines on Biomedical Research Involving Human Subjects. New Delhi, Indian Council of Medical Research, 1997

Indian Psychiatric Society: Ethical Guidelines for Psychiatrists. Cuttack, India, Indian Psychiatric Society, 1989

Reddy GNN: Hinduism and Quality of Life (WHO/MSA/MHP/98.2). Geneva, World Health Organization, 1998

Srinivasa Murthy R: Economics of mental health care in developing countries, in International Review of Psychiatry, Vol 2. Edited by Mack L, Nadelson CC. Washington, DC, American Psychiatric Press, 1996, pp 43–62

Sullivan LE: Healing and Restoring: Health and Medicine in the World's Religious Traditions. New York, Macmillan, 1989

Weiss M: Hinduism, in Encyclopedia of Bioethics, Vol 2. Edited by Reich WT. New York, Macmillan, 1994, pp 1132–1139

Wig NN: Mental health and spiritual values: a view from the East. International Review of Psychiatry 11:92–96, 1999

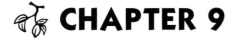

CHAPTER 9

Ethics and Psychiatry in China

Prof. Xiehe Liu

Chinese culture has a long history and is deeply rooted. Traditional Chinese medicine is an essential component of Chinese culture and still has an influence on the Chinese people, especially in rural areas. To describe sufferings in their daily lives, the Chinese often use terms from traditional Chinese medicine such as *disharmony of gas and blood, hyperactivity of the heart fire*, and *hypofunctioning of the kidney*. Many people still prefer to treat their diseases using Chinese herbal drugs or acupuncture. They believe that these treatments have some effects on disease and have fewer side effects. They also believe that treatment in traditional medicine is based on the concept of the human body—including the spirit—as a whole, and that such treatment is comprehensive and holistic, whereas Western medicine has only regional effects and involves the treatment of symptoms. To meet the needs of the Chinese people, Chinese dispensaries carry several hundred kinds of pills and extracts of Chinese herbal drugs in classic preparations. In the past, Confucian ethics, which included the concept of benevolence, were looked up to as the norm for physicians' behavior, and physicians were respected as the embodiment of kindness.

Liji, the book of law and regulations in the Zhou dynasty (1100 B.C.) and one of the Five Classics of ancient China, contained provisions for criminal law. In three types of criminal cases—those in which the person did not recognize his or her aberrant behavior as hazardous or in which the person's offense was considered due to negligence or forgetfulness—the penalty was to be mitigated. In another three types of criminal cases—those in which the offender was young and weak, very old, or mentally retarded—the penalty was to be forgiven (X. Liu 1997). The rationale behind these provisions originated from Confucian ethics of forbearance. The concepts of a universal dichotomy into negative and positive and of the existence of five elementary materials—metal, wood, water, fire, and soil—in Confucian philosophy were well integrated into theories of Chinese traditional medicine.

Psychiatry was not treated as a specialty in medicine in traditional Chinese medicine. The Chinese herbal drugs and acupuncture used in general medicine were also used for mental disorders. When electroconvulsive therapy and psychotropic drugs were introduced in China in the 1940s and 1950s, treatment of mental disorders was radically changed and a new era began. Although psychotropic drugs have been widely used for treating patients with mental illness in recent years, in some remote places these drugs, and doctors trained in their use, are not available. Traditional Chinese medicine fills a need for psychiatric patients and their families. In consideration of similar conditions in medical care of psychiatric patients and of other patients, the Chinese government persistently pursues a double-system policy: it has been making an effort to unite traditional practitioners and practitioners of Western medicine in medical care delivery since 1950. In China from the 1950s to the 1970s, mental disorders were treated with a variety of Chinese herbal drugs, classic and modern prescriptions, and acupuncture, but only a few good results were reported.

Psychiatry in Traditional Chinese Medicine

Descriptions of mental symptoms and mental disorders appeared in the famous Five Classics *(Shi, Shu, Yi, Liji,* and *Chunqiu)* and in the ancient Chinese medical classics (X. Liu 1981). *The Canon of Internal Medicine* was the first medical book of ancient China; it is thought to have been compiled between 300 and 100 B.C. X. Liu (1981) quoted an interesting description of a typical manic state from this book:

> Before the appearance of Kuang [psychosis with excitation], the patient grieves on his own at first. . . . At the beginning of Kuang, the patient feels no hunger. He is in a state of self-praise and self-importance, a self-proclaimed genius. He curses day and night. (X. Liu 1981, p. 430)

In earlier times, the features of manic episodes were prominent and not very different from those seen at present. The cause of this condition was supposed to be the fire. *The Canon of Internal Medicine* stated that "all Kuang and excitement originated from the fire" (C. Liu et al. 1964, p. 8) As a rule, prescription drugs with laxative action for clearing the heat and eliminating the fire were used for these patients (C. Liu et al. 1964). The fire and the heat were thought to be the cause of diseases with symptoms of hyperfunctioning.

A variety of abnormal behaviors in mentally ill patients were described in *The Valuable Prescriptions*, an encyclopedia of medical treatment compiled by the famous physician Sun Simiao (560?–682 A.D.). C. Liu et al. (1964) quoted from this work as follows:

> The patient sometimes keeps silent without voice and sometimes talks a lot rudely; sometimes, he sings and cries and sometimes, chants and laughs; sometimes, he sits and lies in a ditch and eats dirty things, but sometimes he wanders naked day and night; sometimes he curses endlessly; and sometimes he appears with shaky hands and startling eyes, as if he was bewitched by the spirit. (C. Liu et al. 1964, p. 9 [my translation])

This disturbed behavior could be seen in chronic schizophrenia anywhere, before psychotropic drugs were introduced. In ancient times, these patients were considered to have *dian* (psychosis without excitation) and the supposed cause was obstruction of heart orifices by sputum. Herbal drugs for the induction of vomiting were used to expel sputum and reopen the orifices.

The term *zhanwang* (delirium) repeatedly appeared in *The Canon of Internal Medicine* (Y. Xu 1955). Y. Xu (1955) quoted the book's description of this state:

> Water in this year was overwhelming and cold air was prevailing. As evil encroached the heart fire, people suffered from body fever. They became frigid and felt palpitation. . . . The delirium appeared after catching cold. (Y. Xu 1955, p. 169 [my translation])

Delirium was even more frequently mentioned in Zhang Zhongjing's classic book, *On Suffering From Cold*. Zhang Zhongjing, the Hippocrates of China, was born at the beginning of the second century. After an epidemic of infectious disease, he wrote the book to summarize his experiences in clinical practice. "Suffering from cold" was supposed to be the cause of the infectious disease, and then the phrase was used in the title of his book. In this work, he described the diurnal alteration of consciousness in delirious patients (quoted in Y. Xu 1955):

In a woman suffering from cold and having fever, her consciousness was clear during the daytime, and delirious in the evening as seeing ghosts. (Y. Xu 1955, p. 170 [my translation])

Descriptions of nearly 300 herbal preparations for treatment of infectious diseases were collected in this book.

Symptoms of other mental disorders, such as epileptic seizures, hysterical possessed state, globus hystericus, and postpartum psychosis, were also described in the ancient Chinese medical books (X. Liu 1981). There do not appear to be many differences between the basic features of mental disorders in ancient China and those in modern China, nor between such features in Western countries and those in Eastern countries. However, interpretations of etiology and pathogenesis of mental disorders and their treatment differ and have depended on ideology and culture. The ideology of traditional Chinese medicine was based on ancient Chinese philosophy. Mental disorders were thought to be diseases of the heart, kidney, and brain. They were attributed to evil winds, fire, sputum, sluggish gas and stagnant blood, or emotional factors. Diagnosis involved a standardized approach: *liujing bianzheng*, *bagang bianzheng*, *zangfu bianzheng*, and *yingweiqixue bianzheng* (identification of the symptom complex according to six channels, eight outlines, viscera, and barrier-defense-gas-blood, respectively). General rules for treating mental disorders—*qingre xiehuo* (clearing the heat and eliminating the fire), *ditan kaiqiao* (expelling sputum and reopening obstructed orifices), *liqi huoxue* (regulating sluggish gas and activating stagnant blood), and *wenyang bushen* (stimulating the positive function of the body and recruiting the kidney)—were directly related to the mental symptoms. Given the influence of this ancient ideology, it is perhaps not surprising that psychiatry was underdeveloped in traditional Chinese medicine.

Influence of Culture on Modern Psychiatry

Near the end of the nineteenth century, communication between the West and the East was facilitated and cultural exchanges became more frequent. More missionaries and physicians from Western countries came to China. They introduced their religion or fields of medicine and science to the Chinese people. At the same time, a small number of young students were sent abroad to study Western philosophy, ethics, literature, art, medicine, and science. In 1898 the American doctor John G. Kerr established the first institution for the mentally ill in China (Selden 1908). After that, asylums were set up in Beijing (in 1906), Chengdu (in 1909), Harbin (in 1910), Shenyang (in 1914), Suzhou (in 1923), Shanghai (in 1935), Dalian (in 1935), and Nanjing (in 1947) (T. Xu 1995; Y. Xu and Liu 1981). The asylum in Harbin was established by a Russian railway company, and those in Shenyang and Dalian were established by the Japanese. In Suzhou, a ward for mentally ill patients opened in an American Christian hospital. In psychiatric hospitals in Shanghai, the Austrian physician F. Halpern was invited to be director or a consultant (T. Xu 1995).

In the early twentieth century, several medical schools or colleges were established in China and a number of Western physicians were invited to be professors there. Neurology and psychiatry were taught in these medical colleges. The first generation of Chinese neuropsychiatrists was trained at the Peking Union Medical College by American professors A. H. Woods and R. S. Lyman in the 1930s. A few were trained in Shenyang by Japanese professors. Afterward, most of these Chinese neuropsychiatrists went abroad to gain clinical experience in different countries with different cultures, such as the United States, the United Kingdom, France, Canada, and Japan. In the 1940s, when they returned from abroad, electroconvulsive therapy and insulin coma therapy were brought to China.

In the 1950s, a great deal of social change occurred in China. The number of psychiatric hospitals increased rapidly. Most provinces have one or more hospitals for care of mentally ill patients. In Nanjing, Shanghai, Changsha, Beijing, and Chengdu, several training centers for modern psychiatrists gradually developed under the supervision of the first generation of Chinese psychiatrists. By order of the government, every specialty, including psychiatry, was taught from materials from the former Soviet Union. Textbooks of clinical psychiatry, child psychiatry, and forensic psychiatry were translated into Chinese.

The Soviet physiologist Pavlov's theories of conditioned reflex had to be learned by doctors, nurses, teachers, and students in medical colleges. During this period, Soviet culture had a great influence on the Chinese people. Aspects of Western psychology and psychotherapy, such as Freudian psychoanalysis and Adolf Meyer's psychobiology, were considered reactionary and were not taught. However, in the late 1950s, psychotropic drugs were imported from Western countries, which pushed Chinese modern psychiatry into a new era.

The period from 1966 to 1978 was a time of upheaval for the Chinese people. Skepticism was advocated in political movements as well as in the academic field. In psychiatry, electroconvulsive therapy, insulin coma therapy, and drug therapy with large doses were criticized by a small number of youths as instruments of the bourgeois dictatorship against the proletariat. Traditional Chinese medicine, acupuncture, and the doctrines of Chairman Mao were to be used in the treatment of mentally ill patients instead. During this period, preparations of Chinese herbal drugs and electric acupuncture were used on a large scale in psychiatric practice. Some enthusiastic young doctors lived and ate together with the mentally ill patients and attempted to persuade the patients to give up their hallucinations, delusions, and catatonic stupor by showing them the facts and by education. Miracles did not occur. The development of modern Chinese psychiatry restarted after this period of political turmoil ended in the late 1970s.

In the early 1980s, a national epidemiological survey of mental disorders was carried out in 12 regions in China under the direction of World Health Organization consultants. After this study, workshops related to psychiatry and mental health and supported by the World Health Organization were held in different places in China. Social psychiatry and transcultural psychiatry in China developed rapidly. Training programs for master's degrees and doctorates in several medical universities greatly improved the quality of medical education and research. Starting in 1978, the number of international academic exchanges increased more quickly. More and more postgraduate students and young psychiatrists were sent abroad. They brought new techniques and new ideas back to China and moved modern Chinese psychiatry to a new level.

In the 1990s, more laboratories for the biological study of mental disorders were opened. International collaborative research groups are now very active. A number of large pharmaceutical companies entered the Chinese market, which accelerated the use of new drugs in clinical practice and promoted international academic exchange in psychiatry. In addition, psychotherapy and psychological counseling are now more commonly used when needed. A comprehensive specialty of psychiatry has been formed in China as a result of exchanges between Eastern and Western cultures.

Influence of Culture on Mental Disorders

Selden (1937) wrote that "mental diseases occur among the Chinese [that are] very similar to those found among Western peoples. The . . . treatment is [as] efficient [as] in Western lands" (p. 707). It is true that the basic features of mental disorders do not differ much among persons with mental illness in different countries. This general observation is the theoretical foundation for international classification of mental disorders. It is also true that the basic features of mental disorders have not changed much in the last 60 years. However, cultures do have an important influence on some mental disorders. *Koro* is a well-known example. It was suggested that *koro* is a culture-bound psychogenic disorder and that the Chinese are particularly vulnerable. There were several epidemics in southeastern countries and in southern China. In the latest epidemic in Hainan (in southern China), in 1984–1985, about 3,000–4,000 individuals were affected. A popular belief among the people in these areas was that if the penis shrank into the abdomen, the person would die. This belief can be traced to a statement in *The Canon of Internal Medicine:* "Yang [here indicates penis] shrank into the abdomen, which suggests the patient was incurable" (quoted in Mo 1991, p. 2). The belief was thought to play an important role in the outbreak of *koro* (Mo 1991).

Another example of cultural influence on mental disorders is the mental disorders induced by Q*igong.* This ancient exercise includes breathing modulation and meditation and has been popularly practiced for general health for thousands of years. Relatively recently, Q*igong* was said to have the power to cure a variety of chronic diseases. As a result, thousands and thousands of people practiced this exercise during a short period in the 1980s. Since 1985, more than 600 cases of psychosis or neurosis induced by Q*igong* during the exercise have been reported (Bai et al. 1997; Shan et al. 1987). As found in follow-up studies, prognosis in most cases has been good. The psychogenesis might be related to disturbance of autosuggestion during the meditation stage.

A series of social changes have occurred in China since 1949 that have had important effects on the spectrum of mental disorders. In the early 1950s, prostitution and drug abuse were forbidden by the central government. Prostitutes and drug addicts were institutionalized. As a result, general paresis (i.e., dementia from syphilis) and drug abuse disappeared rapidly. At that time, the prevailing diagnosis of mental disorders was neurasthenia. Any patients who had tension headaches or insomnia without physical illness or major mental disease were considered to have neurasthenia. The conditions of this heterogeneous group of patients included chronic fatigue caused by a long history of overwork, neurotic depression, primary insomnia, generalized anxiety, and somatoform disorders. In the 1950s, political movements occurred one after another. The Chinese were encouraged to put all their strength into their work. Chronic fatigue due to overwork was a common phenomenon, and tension headaches and insomnia were frequent complaints. In the 1960s, especially during the Cultural Revolution, people were motivated to participate in political movements. During these movements, regular work was neglected in most circumstances and enthusiasm for the movement replaced dedication to hard work. Gradually, the number of neurasthenic patients greatly decreased in outpatient departments. At the end of 1970s, the *International Classification of Diseases*, 9th Revision (ICD-9) (World Health Organization 1977) was introduced in China. Its classification of neuroses was used instead of the old diagnostic triumvirate (neurasthenia, hysteria, and psychasthenia or obsessive-compulsive neurosis). Depressive neurosis and anxiety neurosis were differentiated from neurasthenia, and phobic neurosis was differentiated from obsessive-compulsive neurosis. However, patients with chronic asthenic syndrome of unknown cause are still considered to have neurasthenia. In an epidemiological survey on neuroses in seven areas of China in 1993, the prevalence of neurasthenia was found to be 8.39 per 1,000 population, the prevalence of depressive neurosis was 3.02 per 1,000, and the prevalence of hysteria was 1.34 per 1,000 (Li et al. 1998). The estimated prevalence of neurasthenia in 1959 was 5.9 per 1,000 population (X. Liu 1992), a figure significantly less than the 1993 prevalence of 8.39 per 1,000.

The turmoil of the Cultural Revolution settled in 1976. Economic reform then began in China. The social lives of the Chinese people have improved greatly since then. However, after the social changes, alcohol consumption greatly increased and the prevalence of alcohol dependence also increased rapidly, as shown in Table 9–1. The prevalence was much higher in minority areas (3.03–43.09 per 1,000) than in Han areas (0.21–6.61 per 1,000); was much higher among people who performed heavy physical labor (68.89 per 1,000) than among office workers (17.69–24.91 per 1,000); and was much higher among people with low incomes (56.25 per 1,000) than among those with high incomes (15.03 per 1,000) (Shen 1987; Shen et al. 1992). It seems that the increase in prevalence of alcohol dependence was correlated not

TABLE 9–1.   Prevalence of alcohol dependence in China

Year	Type or location of survey	Prevalence rate (per 1,000)
1982	Collaborative survey	0.19
1984	Shandong	0.31–0.37
1986	Chongqing	4.55
1986	Hubei	0.33–6.61
1992	Collaborative study	37.27[a]

[a]The average prevalence rates were 57.87 per 1,000 among males and 0.91 per 1,000 among females.
Source. X. Liu 1994; Shen et al. 1992.

with increased income but rather with increased alcohol production and the consequent greater availability.

Another severe social problem in the 1990s was drug abuse. Heroin abuse reappeared in China during the late 1980s, and its prevalence has increased rapidly since that time. Lifetime prevalence of illicit drug use in five high-risk areas in China (Guizhou, Guangzhou, Lanzhou, Yunnan, and Xian) in 1993 was 1.08 per 1,000 population (Xiao et al. 1996). More and more people living in other areas have been affected. In Chengdu, the prevalence was 0.5 per 1,000 in 1994 (Hu et al. 1996), similar to the average prevalence across China according to the Minister of Public Health.

As a result of the improvement of public health and the increase in average life span in the Chinese population, the prevalence of senile dementia has increased during recent decades. At various times during the 1980s, the prevalence of senile dementia was reported as 7.54, 8.1, and 38.67 per 1,000 (Chen et al. 1992). In a 1998 epidemiological survey of 5,225 subjects more than 55 years old carried out by X. Liu et al. (1999) in the Chengdu area, the prevalence of senile dementia was found to be 25.8 per 1,000. Among this population, the prevalence of Alzheimer's disease was 21.1 per 1,000 and that of vascular dementia was 3.4 per 1,000. The prevalence increased rapidly in the group of individuals who were older than 70 years.

The prevalences of schizophrenia and affective disorders seem not to be affected by social changes. Prevalences determined in two collaborative epidemiological surveys carried out in China in 1982 and 1993 are compared in Table 9–2.

The slight increase in prevalence of both schizophrenia and affective disorders might be explained by the increase in patient life expectancy. The prevalence of affective disorders in China was lower than in other countries. Differences in survey methodology are not the sole cause; rather, social or cultural differences should be considered.

TABLE 9–2.   Prevalences of schizophrenia and affective disorders

	Prevalence of schizophrenia (per 1,000)		Prevalence of affective disorders (per 1,000)	
Year of survey	Point	Lifetime	Point	Lifetime
1982	4.75	5.69	0.37	0.76
1993	5.31	6.55	0.52	0.83

Note.   P > .05.
Source.   Chen et al. 1998; J. Wang et al. 1998.

Culture and Psychiatric Services

In China, mentally ill patients and their families can choose between psychiatrists, general practitioners, traditional Chinese healers, witch doctors, and Qigong trainers. Because of stigma, psychiatrists are not the first choice of patients and their families seeking help. When patients or their families are obliged to enter a psychiatric hospital, they look around to be sure no one they know sees them. In consideration of this, some psychiatric hospitals in the past used serial numbers followed by the word *hospital* as their names, and there is talk of changing the title of departments of psychiatry in general hospitals to "Department of Psychological Counseling" or "Ward of Psychosomatic Disease." However, most large psychiatric hospitals are now called mental health centers. In rural areas, psychiatrists are usually not available, and general practitioners or traditional Chinese healers are often patients' first choice. Poor families who cannot afford medical treatment might choose witch doctors. In a survey of the treatment of schizophrenia in northeastern China, it was found that 60.5% of patients were first treated with witchcraft (S. Wang et al. 1997). A survey on help-seeking behavior in a county showed that 63.4% of neurotic patients went to see general practitioners first, 28.6% visited private clinics first, and only 8.0% went to psychiatric clinics first (Zheng and Yao 1997). Some chronic neurotic patients may seek help from traditional Chinese healers or Qigong trainers in other cities.

Before 1950, there were about 10 psychiatric hospitals—with 1,100 beds for psychiatric patients—for 400 million people. By 1990, the number of psychiatric hospitals had increased to 803 (X. Liu 1994), with concomitant increases in the number of beds for psychiatric patients (Table 9–3). Beds for psychiatric patients made up a slightly increased percentage of all hospital beds over this period. At the same time, the number of psychiatrists also increased rapidly (Table 9–4).

The rapid increase in the number of psychiatric facilities and personnel was in response to the urgent need for psychiatric services. In addition to the limited number of psychiatric hospitals set up by public health authorities, more psychiatric hospitals were established by civil administration departments, industry, railway companies, and military organizations. In the late 1980s, the department of public security began to set up security hospitals for criminal offenders with mental disorders. Some private psychiatric hospitals have also been established since then. However, the numbers of beds for psychiatric patients per 100,000 population (8.2) and psychiatrists per 100,000 population (1.02) in China in 1990 were still much lower than those in more developed countries (Desjarlais et al. 1995). The population in

TABLE 9—3.   Numbers of hospital beds and beds for psychiatric
patients in China

Year	No. of beds for psychiatric patients	Total no. of hospital beds	No. of beds for psychiatric patients/total no. of hospital beds (%)
1963	18,776	544,307	3.4
1978	45,269	1,092,914	4.1
1985	71,984	1,487,148	4.8
1990	93,471	1,847,072	5.1

Source.   Ministry of Public Health 1992.

TABLE 9—4.   Numbers of psychiatrists in China

Year	No. of psychiatrists
1950	<100
1963	1,404
1978	3,128
1985	6,683
1990	11,570

Source.   X. Liu 1994.

China in 1990 was 1,133.7 million. However, because of inflation of medical costs, which had begun by the end of the 1980s, the number of beds for psychiatric patients was relatively in excess. The rate of occupancy of beds for psychiatric patients in most psychiatric hospitals decreased from 95% in the 1980s to 60%–80% in the 1990s.

Community-based psychiatric services are not popular in China, except in a few large cities such as Shanghai and Beijing and in some rural areas in Shandong and Sichuan. Most mentally ill persons who cannot afford medical treatment are cared for by their families. Family bonds are still very strong in modern China. Family members usually feel strongly responsible for taking care of sick individuals in their families. Multiple-step regression analysis showed that family care was the most influential factor in prognosis in chronic schizophrenia (Li et al. 1987).

Many patients treated with psychotropic drugs take their medicine irregularly. Compliance rates in two studies involving schizophrenic patients were

67.5%–75.3% (Jiang et al. 1997; L. Xu et al. 1987). In the noncompliance group, the relapse rate was very high and the prognosis was rather poor. Usually more than 50% of beds for psychiatric patients are occupied by readmitted patients. In a country with limited psychiatric resources, this is a huge waste. To improve the use of medical resources in China, psychosocial education of relatives of schizophrenic patients has been carried out in some communities, with good results (Zhang et al. 1998). Education of these patients and of general practitioners about psychotropic drugs is also important for reducing relapse rates and improving prognosis.

Other Issues

In the 1950s, a number of psychiatric hospitals were set up by civil administration departments in most provinces for admission of homeless patients, who were treated free of charge. In 1958, the first national conference on prevention and treatment of mental disorders was held in Nanjing. At this conference, physical restraint of mentally ill patients was criticized and active treatment was advocated.

Conclusions

The long history of the development of Chinese psychiatry can be divided into two parts: before the twentieth century and after the twentieth century. Before the twentieth century, psychiatry was not a specialty but one part of the general traditional Chinese medicine. Theories and clinical practice of psychiatry were mainly influenced by traditional Chinese ethics and philosophy. During the twentieth century, under the influence of Western medicine and culture, psychiatry developed as a comprehensive modern psychological medicine.

References

Bai L, Wang Y, Hou R: *Qigong* induced mental disorders: follow-up study of 29 cases [in Chinese]. Chinese Mental Health Journal 11:357, 1997

Chen C, Shen Y, Li S, et al: An epidemiological survey on dementia in an aged population in the western urban district of Beijing [in Chinese]. Chinese Journal of Mental Health 6:49–52, 1992

Chen C, Shen Y, Li S, et al: Epidemiological survey on schizophrenia in 7 areas of China [in Chinese]. Chinese Journal of Psychiatry 31:72–74, 1998

Desjarlais R, Eisenberg L, Good B, et al: World Mental Health: Problems and Priorities in Low-Income Countries. New York, Oxford University Press, 1995, p 56

Hu Z, Liu X, He K, et al: A survey on prevalence of drug abuse in five urban areas of Chengdu City [in Chinese]. Chinese Journal of Behavioral Medical Science 5: 138–139, 1996

Jiang K, Li S, Lo X, et al: Compliance in schizophrenic maintenance treatment [in Chinese]. Chinese Journal of Psychiatry 30:167–170, 1997

Li S, Chen C, Zhang W: A computer analysis of multiple step regression for the possible factors contributing to the prognosis of schizophrenia [in Chinese]. Chinese Mental Health Journal 1:180–182, 1987

Li S, Shen Y, Zhang W, et al: Epidemiological survey on neuroses [in Chinese]. Chinese Journal of Psychiatry 31:80, 1998

Liu C, He M, Xiang M, et al: Introdution, in Psychiatry, 2nd Edition. Edited by Liu C, He M, Xiang M, et al. Beijing, People's Medical Publishing House, 1964, pp 5–14

Liu X: Psychiatry in traditional Chinese medicine. Br J Psychiatry 138:429–433, 1981

Liu X: Neurasthenia, in Chinese Medical Encyclopedia. Edited by Qian X (Editor in Chief). Shanghai, Shanghai Science and Technology Publishing House, 1992, pp 75–76

Liu X: Our mental health services today and tomorrow. Paper presented at a meeting of the Royal Society of Medicine, Section of Psychiatry, London, England, May 10, 1994

Liu X: Introduction, in Forensic Psychiatry. Edited by Liu X. Beijing, People's Medical Publishing House, 1997, pp 1–5

Liu X, Tang M, Zhou X, et al: An epidemiological study on senile dementia in Chengdu area, China [in Chinese]. Paper presented at the VIII Congress of the International Federation of Psychiatric Epidemiology, Taipei, China, March 6–9, 1999

Ministry of Public Health: Year Book of Health in the People's Republic of China 1991. Beijing, The People's Medical Publishing House, 1992

Mo G: Introduction, in Epidemic Koro. Edited by Mo G. Guangzhou, China, Guangdong Science and Technology Publishing House, 1991, pp 1–8

Selden CC: The John G. Kerr Refuge for the Insane. Chin Med J 22:82–91, 1908

Selden CC: The story of the John G. Kerr Hospital for the Insane. Chin Med J 52:707–714, 1937

Shan H, Yan H, Xu S, et al: A study of clinical phenomenology on mental disorders caused by breathing exercise [in Chinese]. Chinese Journal of Nervous and Mental Disease 13:266–269, 1987

Shen Y: Recent epidemiological data on alcoholism in China [in Chinese]. Chinese Mental Health Journal 1:251–252, 256, 1987

Shen Y, Zhang W, Lu Q, et al: Epidemiological survey on alcohol dependence in populations of four occupations in nine cities of China, I: methodology and prevalence [in Chinese]. Chinese Mental Health Journal 6:112–115, 1992

Wang J, Wang D, Shen Y, et al: Epidemiological survey on affective disorder in 7 areas of China [in Chinese]. Chinese Journal of Psychiatry 31:75–77, 1998

Wang S, Qi F, Guo Y, et al: A survey on pre-admission treatment of schizophrenic patients [in Chinese]. Chinese Mental Health Journal 11:189, 1997

World Health Organization: International Classification of Diseases, 9th Revision. Geneva, World Health Organization, 1977

Xiao S, Hao W, Yang D: Epidemiological study on illicit drug use in five high risk areas of China, I: lifetime prevalence of illicit drug use [in Chinese]. Chinese Mental Health Journal 10:234–238, 1996

Xu L, Wang J, Wang Q, et al: Evaluation of persistent or interrupted treatment for schizophrenics [in Chinese]. Chinese Journal of Neurology and Psychiatry 19: 175–178, 1986

Xu T: History of the development of modern Chinese psychiatry, in On the Development of Modern Chinese Neurology and Psychiatry [in Chinese]. Edited by Chen Xueshi, Chen Xiuhua. Beijing, Chinese Science and Technology Publishing House, 1995, pp 6–17

Xu Y: Psychiatry in ancient China [in Chinese]. Chinese Journal of Neurology and Psychiatry 1:167–174, 1955

Xu Y, Liu X: History of psychiatry, in Foundations of Psychological Medicine, Vol 1. Edited by Hunan Medical College. Changsha, China, Hunan Science and Technology Publishing House, 1981, pp 1–32

Zhang M, Weng Z, Yan H, et al: Two-year experience of psychosocial education for relatives of schizophrenics [in Chinese]. Chinese Journal of Psychiatry 31:90–93, 1998

Zheng C, Yao Z: A survey on help-seeking behavior of neurotic patients [in Chinese]. Chinese Mental Health Journal 11:190, 1997

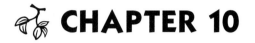 CHAPTER 10

Intersubjectivity and Its Influence on Psychiatry in Japan

Prof. Yoshibumi Nakane
Prof. Mark Radford

If my heart just follows the Way, the gods will watch over me even though I neglect to pray to them.

> Sugawara no Michizane,
> poet-scholar (Heian period [794–1185])

In the West, *ethics* relates to individuality or subjectivity. The English word *ethics* derives ultimately from the Greek word *ethos*, which means "custom" or "character." Ethics are the principles that govern human nature.

Japanese ethics, on the other hand, has been described as unique. It is "merely a pattern of social living. . . . It is realistic, almost opportunistic, apparently without absolutes or universals, except for the one basic ethical principle of duty-loyalty to the group and to the superior-dominated and exclusively Japanese social nexus—and whatever actions are required thereby" (Moore 1967, p. 297). For Japanese, the study of ethics is the study of intersubjectivity, or the principles that guide the behavior between people within a community. *Rinrigaku*, the Japanese literal translation of *ethics*, refers to the principles that exist between human beings.

This chapter is divided into three major sections. In the first section, we briefly examine the meaning of ethics in Japan and look at some of the concepts associated with Japanese ethics. In the second section, we focus on the relationship between ethics and medicine. In the third and final section, we look at how the definition of ethics has changed to include the concept of human rights, and we examine the role of human rights in medicine, especially in psychiatric care, and associated changes in legislation.

Japanese Ethics

The Japanese approach to human existence has strong roots in Chinese philosophical thought, especially Confucianism. Buddhism also has had an impact. Although it is not possible to discuss Japanese ethics in detail here, it is helpful to identify some important elements.

The importance of intersubjectivity to an understanding of Japanese thinking and behavior is reflected in the number of works published in Japanese and other languages on the topic. The notion that the individual is inseparable from his or her status within the community is an important one in Japan. Some writers have even gone to the extent of saying that Japanese are devoid of self-consciousness (Inatomi 1963). Although this may be a somewhat extreme view, it is true that self-consciousness is often defined and seen in terms of its relationship to "social consciousness."

In Japanese society, the thinking and behavior that make up the social consciousness involve maintaining the social order. The mechanisms at the heart of maintaining the social order are social harmony *(wa)* and social obligation (e.g., *giri)*.

Wa is not simply "mechanical cooperation, starting from reasons, of equal individuals independent of each other, but the grand harmony *(taiwa)* which maintains its integrity by proper statuses of individuals within the collectivity and by acts in accordance with these statuses" (Mobusho 1937, p. 51 [translated by Kawashima 1967]). *Wa* means a number of things—harmony, conciliation, reconciliation, submission, and unity. Although autonomous decision-making can occur, many decisions of consequence are made in reference to the immediate social group (e.g., family, social club members, or colleagues). Such decision making ensures the maintenance of *wa* (Radford and Nakane 1991).

In Japanese culture, as in most cultures, there is a strong respect for human life. In Confucianism, one is taught about the virtue of *jin* (from the Chinese, meaning "human heartedness"). Buddhism stresses the importance of *jihi* (mercy). Relationships between people involve some form of social obligation (e.g., *giri)*. In Japan, social obligation is seen as a voluntary act on the part of the individual under that obligation and involves a strong element of "added" indebtedness.

In Japanese society, the concept of equality between human beings, though not unknown, is understood differently than in the West. In Japan, although the individual is often seen as having a wide range of nuances and attributes, as "a discrete entity with its own status and value" (Kawashima 1967, p. 263), he or she is nevertheless subject to the corporate view. However, this conception often entails a belief that the individual cannot be seen as equal to others, simply because he or she is independent. Everyone has their own roles based on these nuances and attributes and based on the context in which they find themselves. "In a society with such assumptions, laws and ethics aim at maintaining the social order consisting in the statuses of men with immense variety as they actually exist and not at imposing a social order which is postulated by intellect or ideal" (Kawashima 1967, p. 263).

At the individual level, there has long been an assumption that the individual needs to be submissive to authority (Minami 1971). This assumption has been described as essential for an understanding of Japanese thought and interpersonal relationships. *Giri*, mentioned earlier, dictates a certain attitude and behavior toward those people who are a part of one's social network. *Giri* helps to maintain the social order, relationships, and interdependency *(amae)* between people.

Amae refers to the desire to be close to others and the need to depend on others for support. As a trait, it is considered to be an important key for understanding the Japanese psyche (Doi 1981). As a concept, *amae* refers to relationships between people that are similar to a child's feeling for his or her parents (especially the mother). *Amae* in interpersonal relationships is the basis of hierarchical relationships in Japanese society. "In such relationships, one person, usually the younger or junior, is dependent on the other, usually the senior. *Amae* is seen in most formal relationships in Japan—including the relationship between . . . doctor and patient" (Radford and Nakane 1999, p. 213).

The importance placed on *wa*, the *amae* personality, and social obligation has given rise to the notion that Japanese are imbued with the "spirit of the governed" (which prevents individuals from exercising rights and performing duties as autonomous individuals) and the "spirit of the taught" (which refers to a passive attitude with respect to authority) (see Minami 1971 and Furukawa 1967).

It can be argued that these two "spirits," combined with a natural tendency to depend on others for help, can create an environment in which the rights of patients can be overlooked to protect the community as a whole. Authority figures (including doctors) have the right and in many cases are expected to make decisions on behalf of the patient with the good of both the patient and the community in mind.

Ethics and Medicine

Our understanding of the individual and the individual's relationship with his or her environment is dependent on existing ethical and moral standards. These standards have an important influence on the way we understand, interpret, and react to the different situations with which we are faced during life. The practice of medicine is no exception.

In Japan, most patients think they are asking their doctors a favor when they present with medical problems. They tend not to question the decisions that doctors make. As one writer put it, "They . . . try to be as good and obedient a patient as possible . . . [and generally] do not care much about their civil rights" (Hoshino 1997, p. 14). Some patients even go as far as rejecting attempts by physicians to explain medical conditions and treatments, believing that they should not be burdened by such information and decision-making—those are the doctor's responsibility. Hoshino (1997) linked this attitude to the Japanese proverb "manaita no ue no koi," which means that a patient is resigned to his or her fate—the patient autonomously resigns himself or herself to the physician's care.

Family responsibility for looking after ill family members means that traditionally, medical decisions are made in consultation with family members and not by the patient alone. Care for a patient is often provided by a family member (usually female); and even when the patient must stay in the hospital, it is not unusual for a family member to stay overnight. As the onus on the family becomes greater, family members often talk directly with doctors about the patient's condition, obtaining information without the consent of the patient. As mentioned earlier, the notion that an individual has rights outside his or her social context (i.e., the family) is relatively unknown in Japan.

This situation is especially true in the medical setting. With family responsibility comes the perception that it is the family's duty to obtain the required information. Often the truth about certain diagnoses, such as cancer, is not revealed to patients, with more than 90% of doctors hiding the diagnosis from their patients (Mizushima et al. 1990). "This duty is perceived without any thought that they might be infringing upon the patient's right to autonomy, self-determination and privacy. There is, in fact, no concept in the mind of the Japanese that one of the family members has such individual rights independent of the family" (Hoshino 1997, p. 17).

Recent studies suggest, however, that although provision of information to patients is still regarded as being at the discretion of the physician, more and more doctors are willing to give their patients sufficient information for them to give informed consent to treatment (Hattori et al. 1991; Kai et al. 1993; for an extensive discussion see Beauchamp 1997).

National Legislation and Mental Health Care

In Western societies, there is a belief that each human being has certain rights that he or she can demand or expect others to respect and even protect. Until the 1860s (the beginning of the Meiji era), this concept of human rights was not a part of Japanese thinking. However, soon after the Meiji restoration, the notion of human rights was introduced into Japan. Although the idea gained acceptability, it was not until after World War II that it was widely accepted. (For a fuller discussion, see Kawashima 1967.)

With the introduction of the concept of human rights, as well as in response to the changing nature of psychiatric thought and practice in Japan, the concept of welfare has become a fundamental part of psychiatric care. It was incorporated within national legislation in 1900 when the Diet (Japanese parliament) passed the Confinement and Protection for Lunatics Act. This act was revised in 1919 and renamed the Mental Hospital Act. This legislation lasted until 1950, when the Mental Hygiene Law was passed, with a partial revision being made in 1965. In 1987, the Mental Hygiene Law was replaced by the Mental Health Law, which itself was revised in 1993.

In 1995, there was a third major revision and the name was changed to the Law Concerning Mental Health and the Welfare of Those With Mental Disabilities (or the Mental Health Welfare Law) (Ministry of Health and Welfare 1995a). The new law incorporates the notion of patient rights, with a strong emphasis on promoting independence through rehabilitation. Specifically, the aims of the new law are to ensure adequate medical care and protection of mentally disabled patients with reference to patient rights, to promote social rehabilitation of mentally disabled patients in order to promote patient independence (the ability to support oneself) and participation in social and economic activities, and to preserve and improve the mental health of Japanese citizens in general.

With the establishment of the Basic Law Concerning the Disabled in December 1993, social rehabilitation for physically disabled individuals and social rehabilitation for mentally disabled individuals were considered together.

Today, the number of people receiving some kind of psychiatric care in Japan is about 1.6 million (Fujita 1997). Of these, about 340,000 people receive some form of inpatient care in a psychiatric hospital. In 1993, the prevalence of treated patients per 10,000 people was 128.2, compared with 73.6 in 1973 (Table 10–1). Thus, the prevalence increased significantly. However, this increase is due not to an increase in the number of inpatients (23.5 in 1973 to 26.7 in 1993) but to an increase in the number of outpatients (50.1 to 101.5) (Table 10–1).

In general, it is thought that 30,000 of the patients currently in the hospital system could leave if adequate health and welfare support in the community were available. This indicates the urgent need in Japan to develop a community care system.

In addition to the relative and absolute numbers, the nature of inpatient admission has also changed (Fujita 1997). In recent years, the number of involuntary admissions by the prefectural government (forced hospitalization) has sharply declined. There were more than 76,000 involuntary admissions in 1970, with a rate of involuntary admission of 30%; in 1995, there were fewer than 6,000 involuntary admissions and the rate of involuntary admission was less than 2% (Table 10–2). Further, the bed occupancy rate decreased from 105% in 1970 to 94% in 1995 (Table 10–2). Similarly, the number of admissions for medical care and protection (semiforced hospitalization and hospitalization with family agreement) has also decreased. Most hospitalized cases are now through voluntary admission (hospitalization), which involves patient consent.

Inpatient care itself has also changed (Fujita 1997). The number of patients who were admitted and subsequently discharged in 1974 was about 224,000, whereas by 1993 that number had increased by 1.6 times to about 357,000 (Table 10–3). In 1974, about 229,000 patients were hospitalized during the year and 27.7% of them were discharged within a month, whereas in 1990, about 329,000 patients were hospitalized during the year and 40.0% were discharged within a month (Table 10–3). Thus, the number of short-term hospitalizations has increased.

These three tables thus indicate that although there has been a sharp increase in the number of persons seeking medical and psychiatric help, this seeking of help is much more on a voluntary basis and involves reduced hospital stay. It is clear that as a result of recent changes in legislation (and

TABLE 10–1. Estimated numbers and prevalences of patients receiving care for mental disorders

Year	No. of care-receiving patients (in thousands)			Prevalence of treated patients (per 10,000 population)		
	Inpatients	Outpatients	Total	Inpatients	Outpatients	Total
1973	253.9	541.6	795.5	23.5	50.1	73.6
1983	326.6	880.6	1,207.2	27.3	73.7	101.0
1993	332.6	1,266.1	1,598.7	26.7	101.5	128.2

Source. Fujita 1997.

TABLE 10–2. Numbers of inpatients and involuntary admissions, bed occupancy rates, and rates of involuntary admission

Year	No. of beds	No. of inpatients	Bed occupancy rate (%)	No. of involuntary admissions	Rate of involuntary admission (%)
1970	242,022	253,433	104.7	76,597	30.2
1975	275,468	281,127	102.0	65,571	23.3
1980	304,469	311,584	102.3	47,400	15.2
1985	333,570	339,989	101.9	30,543	9.2
1990	358,251	348,859	97.5	12,572	3.6
1995	362,180	340,785	94.1	5,905	1.7

Source. Fujita 1997.

Table 10—3.   Estimated numbers of patients admitted and then discharged and percentages of discharged patients by length of hospitalization

Year	No. of discharged patients (in thousands)	No. of admitted patients (in thousands)	Percentage of discharged patients, by length of hospitalization		
			<1 month	<6 months	<12 months
1974	224.1	229.1	27.7	70.7	81.5
1983	305.4	308.2	32.8	75.9	85.0
1990	350.4	329.4	40.0	80.0	88.0
1993	356.6	ND	ND	ND	ND

Note.   ND = not determined.
Source.   Fujita 1997.

thinking), trends in "enforced" hospitalization and long-term psychiatric institutional care are themselves changing. Hospitalization now involves greater patient consent. Despite limited resources, community-based care is seen as more desirable than hospital-based care.

Until recent history, laws and statutes were often considered *denka no hato* (a sword handed down within a family as an heirloom) (see Kawashima 1967). In other words, they were seen as symbolic and not necessarily meant to be implemented. Although the Western understanding of ethics and morality has had an impact in Japan in the last few decades, especially in the area of legal practice, this impact has had greater influence in terms of formal laws and practices than on the underlying cultural consciousness, which as a result has led to some degree of tension between the two.

In 1996, the Plan for People With Disabilities was implemented (Ministry of Health and Welfare 1995b). Promotion of social rehabilitation and welfare measures for mentally disabled individuals began, as did establishment of various halfway homes for social rehabilitation and community support activities. According to the new Mental Health Welfare Law, peer review concerning appropriateness of care and protection of the human rights of inpatients is to be conducted regularly. The Psychiatric Review Board organized under this law has been functioning, and inpatient requests for discharge or claims for improvement of patient treatment are being taken into consideration and handled promptly. Unfortunately, it is also true that there are some psychiatric hospitals where patients are still treated inadequately, and we still need to work to improve the situation and to offer more appropriate psychiatric care.

The Mental Health Welfare Law also requires Japanese health institutions to increase the number of care staff sufficiently to allow team care. It is hoped that a range of staff will be fully involved in a course of treatment, from inpatient care to outpatient care—staff such as psychiatrists, nurses, clinical psychologists, psychiatric social workers, and occupational therapists. In some more advanced psychiatric hospitals in Japan, such a cooperative team care system has already been adopted. However, there are not enough trained staff for all psychiatric institutions, and it will take time to implement this team approach more generally. Our hospital (Nagasaki University Hospital) has a sufficient number of psychiatrists to provide care for inpatients, outpatients, and day care patients with help from nurses only. However, because of the government's attempt to decrease the number of workers in national universities, it is impossible for our hospital to employ staff in the relatively new care fields, staff such as social workers, psychologists, and occupational therapists. We are far from the goal of the Mental Health Welfare Law.

Conclusions

As we enter a stage of increasing global interdependence and influence, the need for a common understanding of what is right and what is wrong becomes more important. As people move across our planet and are exposed to different beliefs, thinking, and behavior, greater understanding and a common framework for implementing care become more vital. This is especially true in medicine, in which such aspects as organ transplantation, informed consent, patient rights, and drug and other therapies may involve crossing of geographical boundaries.

References

Beauchamp TL: Comparative studies: Japan and America, in Japanese and Western Bioethics: Studies in Moral Diversity. Edited by Hoshino K. Dordrecht, Kluwer Academic, 1997, pp 25–47

Doi T: The Anatomy of Dependency. Translated by Bestar J. Tokyo, Kodansha International, 1981

Fujita T: Current conditions of rehospitalization, and yearly trends of admission/discharge and therapy-receiving patterns in a national sample [in Japanese]. Tokyo, Japan, Ministry of Education, 1997

Furukawa T: The individual in Japanese ethics, in The Japanese Mind: Essentials of Japanese Philosophy and Culture. Edited by Moore CA. Honolulu, HI, East-West Center Press, 1967, pp 228–244

Hattori H, Salzberg SM, Kiang WP, et al: The patient's right to information in Japan—legal rules and doctor's opinions. Soc Sci Med 32:1007–1016, 1991

Hoshino K: Bioethics in the light of Japanese sentiments, in Japanese and Western Bioethics: Studies in Moral Diversity. Edited by Hoshino K. Dordrecht, Kluwer Academic, 1997, pp 13–23

Inatomi E: Nihonjin to Nihonbunka. Tokyo, Risosha, 1963

Kai I, Ohi G, Yano E, et al: Communication between patients and physicians about terminal care: a survey in Japan. Soc Sci Med 36:1151–1159, 1993

Kawashima T: The status of the individual in the notion of law, right, and social order, in The Japanese Mind: Essentials of Japanese Philosophy and Culture. Edited by Moore CA. Honolulu, HI, East-West Center Press, 1967, pp 262–287

Minami H: The Psychology of the Japanese People. Translated by Ikoma AR. Tokyo, University of Tokyo Press, 1971

Ministry of Health and Welfare: The Confinement and Protection for Lunatics Act [in Japanese]. Tokyo, Japan, Ministry of Health and Welfare, 1900

Ministry of Health and Welfare: The Mental Hospital Act [in Japanese]. Tokyo, Japan, Ministry of Health and Welfare, 1919

Ministry of Health and Welfare: The Mental Hygiene Law [in Japanese]. Tokyo, Japan, Ministry of Health and Welfare, 1950

Ministry of Health and Welfare: The Mental Health Law [in Japanese]. Tokyo, Japan, Ministry of Health and Welfare, 1987

Ministry of Health and Welfare: The Basic Law Concerning the Disabled [in Japanese]. Tokyo, Japan, Ministry of Health and Welfare, 1993

Ministry of Health and Welfare: The Law Concerning Mental Health and the Welfare of Those With Mental Disabilities [in Japanese]. Tokyo, Japan, Ministry of Health and Welfare, 1995a

Ministry of Health and Welfare: The Plan for People With Disabilities: A White Paper on Health and Welfare [in Japanese]. Tokyo, Japan, Ministry of Health and Welfare, 1995b

Mizushima Y, Kashii T, Hoshino K, et al: A survey regarding the disclosure of the diagnosis of cancer in Toyama Prefecture, Japan. Japanese Journal of Medicine 29: 146–155, 1990

Mobusho: Kokutai no hongi. Tokyo, Naikaku-insatsukyoku, 1937

Moore CA: Editor's supplement: the enigmatic Japanese mind, in The Japanese Mind: Essentials of Japanese Philosophy and Culture. Edited by Moore CA. Honolulu, HI, East-West Center Press, 1967, pp 288–313

Radford M, Nakane Y: Ishiketteikoi: hikakubungateki kosatsu. Tokyo, Human TY Publishers, 1991

Radford M, Nakane Y: The Japanese psyche and psychopathology, in Images in Psychiatry: Japan. Edited by Nakane Y, Radford M. Paris, France, NHA Communication, 1999, pp 205–220

SECTION II

Overarching Issues

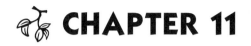

CHAPTER 11

Research Involving
Incompetent Patients

A Current Problem in Light of German History

Prof. Dr. Hanfried Helmchen

Historical Facts and Questions

In the first 30 years after the end of the Third Reich, crimes came to light in Germany that had been committed by the National Socialist German Workers' Party in the name of medicine (Erhardt 1965; Mitscherlich and Mielke 1947, 1960; Schmidt 1965). At that time, these revelations did not bring about a general outcry, doubtless because these atrocities, in which the previous generation was involved to some degree or another, were necessarily regarded as merely the crimes of a few people committed in an exceptional and now-closed chapter in history. The crimes included the following:

♦ *Murder.* Approximately 100,000 persons who were categorized (primarily) as chronically mentally ill were murdered (Finzen 1996).
♦ *Forced sterilization.* More than 300,000 persons underwent forced sterilization, overwhelmingly for eugenic reasons, but for economic reasons as well (Finzen 1996; Meyer-Lindenberg 1991).
♦ *"Scientific" experiments on human beings*, in which death was accepted or intended (Hohendorf et al. 1996; Mitscherlich and Mielke 1960)

This chapter is based on H. Helmchen, "Research With Incompetent Demented Patients." *European Psychiatry* 13 (suppl. 3):93S–100S, 1998.

To the postwar generation, these crimes seemed perforce to have nothing to do with actual medical practice after World War II, and recurrences were regarded as inconceivable. But can we be sure of this in light of developments such as the following:

♦ *Euthanasia* actively practiced on Germany's border in the Netherlands on a large scale and with the growing approval of the population, in cases where no consent was given, and in the case of the mentally ill
♦ *Forced sterilization* practiced in many countries until very recently and particularly in Sweden on a large scale
♦ At the European Union's Convention for the Protection of Human Rights and Dignity as Applied in Biology and Medicine, *study in the human sciences of incompetent persons* was declared permissible in exceptional cases even when no direct benefit would accrue to the persons themselves.

These current developments are of a different quality than the National Socialists' crimes against humanity. However, certain questions must be asked: Which premises underlying these recent developments are comparable and how do they differ from the National Socialist crimes against humanity? What factors led to the transformation of conceptions into criminal acts, not only in National Socialist Germany but in other countries as well? If such mechanisms are known, can preventive measures be determined that could guard against a recurrence of the horrors of the past?

These questions should be answered, using the example of research involving incompetent patients. First, we should make the questions somewhat more concrete to show how difficult it is to draw the line between what is desired and what is dangerous in putting into practice conceptions that are very widespread.

There seems to be no connection between so-called passive euthanasia (denoting the alleviation of the throes of death of a single individual) and the mass murder (designated using the same term) by the National Socialists of mentally ill persons for politico-economic (and in part also scientific) reasons. However, the current discussion of the various forms of "euthanasia" (Helmchen and Vollmann 1999) shows that the number of dying persons who request help in killing themselves (so-called assisted suicide) is growing, that among these persons—as the Chabot case *(State v. Chabot* [1994]) made clear (Fuchs and Lauter 1997; Griffiths 1995)—are mentally ill individuals, and that readiness to end the lives of nondying coma vigil patients by withdrawing nourishment (e.g., the Swiss euthanasia guidelines) appears to be growing. Further, in the Netherlands in 1993, more than 1,000 individuals died as a result of nonvoluntary euthanasia (Fuchs and Lauter 1997).

Voluntary sterilization for the purpose of preventing individual suffering is seemingly worlds apart from forced sterilization for the purpose of "cleansing the body of the people" under National Socialism. Does not the practice of forced sterilization in Sweden, terminated only in 1976, show how thin is the line dividing the welfare state from sinister forms of eugenic-economic social engineering (Burleigh 1994)? In addition to eugenic argumentation, argumentation derived from the socialist *Volksheim* ideology, on the obligatory lowering of societal burdens in financing the welfare state, found its way into the supporting argumentation of the 1935 Swedish sterilization law (von Altenbeckum 1997).

No connection can be discerned between the involvement of a consenting patient in an attempt at healing with potential individual benefit and the killing of nonconsenting children in the name of scientific study by National Socialist doctors (Hohendorf et al. 1996). But reports such as that of Beecher (1966) or Faden (1996) show that even after the adoption of the 1947 Nuremberg Code (Mitscherlich and Mielke 1960), human beings were involved in interventions that purportedly had scientific purposes but that in no way conformed to the code.

Mechanisms That Can Lead to Unethical Behavior

In the past few years, numerous analyses have shown that above all, the following mechanisms made possible the development of "medicine devoid of humanity" (Mitscherlich and Mielke 1960) under the National Socialists (Finzen 1996; Groeben 1990):

- Debasement, systematic denunciation, and degradation of the victims, excluding the victims from the community of human solidarity
- Secretiveness and segregation, preventing checks and control not only by the public but also by state institutions designed to perform monitoring[1]
- Development of group morality, authoritarian obedience, and group pressure
- Coupling of the welfare of society with faith in its instruments of organized violence
- Giving of priority to organizational over individual justification for social acts
- Motivation by higher, national, or social interests

♦ Encouragement of secretive agreement and guilty conscience by appealing to motives that are widespread but mere emotional reflexes (gut reactions)

♦ Prosecution of an ostensibly just cause with fanatical zeal, i.e., investing partial insight with absolute validity

These mechanisms are neither unique nor specific to National Socialism. Both systematic analyses and a plethora of individual experience attest to the fact that many concepts that dominated under National Socialism were and are present in other times and in many other parts of the globe. However, they often existed separately and discretely from one another. Weindling (1985) showed that forced sterilization could be detached from anti-Semitism and "Nordic" ethnocentric racism, that the apologists for forced sterilization did not necessarily support euthanasia,[2] and that social Darwinism was by no means limited to the political right wing (quoted from Burleigh 1997, p. 294).

Each of these individual factors becomes dangerous if it is taken out of its living context (i.e., if it is no longer kept under control by the coexistence of other competing concepts or behavioral attitudes) or if it is invested with absolute validity (i.e., prosecuted to the point of excess). Where does detachment from the social context and the investment of absolute validity begin? In some factors, such as the first two previously mentioned (dehumanization and secretiveness), it—just as in the loss of general acceptance—may be recognizable much sooner than in other factors. Danger is ahead when, under the influence of the social consensus *(zeitgeist)*,[3] the thresholds are shifted and the boundaries disappear. As Mitscherlich and Mielke (1947) formulated in their 1947 report on the Nuremberg Doctors Trial, every physician can become a licensed murderer "when the aggressiveness of his search for the truth intersects the ideology of the dictatorship" (quoted from Hohendorf et al. 1997) (all translations are my own). That is, danger is ahead when ideas are distilled and transformed, when one leaves the world of ideas and enters the material reality of the totalitarian organization of society. Today it seems clear that concepts from individual human experience such as sympathy for those with incurable conditions or those who suffer from afflictions,[4] or the right of individuals to euthanasia[5] based on the principle of individual autonomy, could by virtue of economic necessity[6] or eugenic,[7] socialist,[8] or other ideologies lead to state intervention and, finally, in the totalitarian state form of National Socialism, with its suppression of any and all dissenting public or published opinion *(Gleichschaltung)*, to the destruction of human beings. In recent years, it has been shown how this context indeed led scientifically active physicians to participate in this disastrous development, to gravely violate the principles of physicians, and even to commit crimes.[9]

Because the possibility of such patterns cannot be excluded, whether and how these factors can be kept under reliable control must be determined. Doubts are indeed in order, because even democracy, independent media, and a critical public are not sufficient—or do not appear to be—to prevent the violation of human rights and humanity.[10]

It is decisive that consciousness is sensitized ethically and sensitized effectively so that in borderline cases the physician is capable of weighing competing principles against each other and simultaneously fulfilling his or her medical obligations vis-à-vis the individual patient. Are a few general guidelines, covering even the gray areas, more appropriate in practice? That is, are human dignity and human capacity better taken into account in general guidelines than in detailed procedural instructions?[11] Which approach affords better protection from commission of grave errors and abuse, from taking the first steps toward criminality: denying real dilemmas[12] and investing with absolute validity fundamental principles such as the unquestionable obligation to protect life and the absolute priority of individual rights over community rights; or explicit discussion, weighing the values involved as well as the juridically and legislatively accepted and controllable rules?[13]

A Statement of the German Central Ethics Commission

In Germany, the Central Commission for the Protection of Ethical Principles in Medicine and Related Fields (Central Ethics Commission), independently affiliated with the Federal Chamber of Physicians, decided in favor of the latter approach (explicit discussion) and formulated its position on "the protection of mentally incompetent persons in medical research" (Zentrale Ethikkommission 1997a, pp. B2194–B2196):

> A particular ethical dilemma arises in research, the results of which benefit not the patient involved but other persons in the same age group or with the same illness or disorder. On the one hand, subjecting a person without his or her consent to a measure on behalf of others but which brings no benefit to him or her is prohibited ("prohibition of instrumentalization"). On the other hand, we have the ethical conviction that a person can be subjected to a slight risk if, thereby, great benefit accrues to others. No one—whether he or she is mentally competent or not—can be obligated to participate in a scientific study for the benefit of a future group of patients, even when the benefit for these patients is

considerable and the risks for him or her are minimal. However, the involvement of incompetent persons in such a study appears to be defensible if—apart from observing other protective criteria—the knowledge that the person's legal representative has of him or her (in particular, behavior, attitudes and/or explicit statements in the past) constitutes sufficient grounds to support the conclusion that the person would consent to participation in the study. (Zentrale Ethikkommission 1997a, pp. B2194–B2196).

Thus, the dilemma in this case, arising from competing ethical principles, is clearly set forth, showing the preconditions under which the mandate of rendering assistance through research can be valid not only for this individual patient but for defined groups of patients as well, and thus possibly at the expense (to a defined minimal degree) of the individual patient. In another discussion paper, the Central Ethics Commission (Zentrale Ethikkommission 1997b) called attention to the fact that "even Basic Law as the basis of the individual's right to self-determination does not embody a conception of the human being with individualistic and self-serving ends, to whom any concept whatsoever of solidarity and integration in the social community is alien" (p. A1912).

In contrast,

the Federal Constitutional Court has emphasized repeatedly that Basic Law resolves the tension between the individual and the community in favor of the individual's community orientation and community obligation without calling into question the value of the individual. . . . Therefore, it is not excluded *a priori* that measures can be admissible which are only slightly stressful for the patient involved, even without his or her express consent, if through these measures great benefit accrues to other persons in the same category and if this benefit cannot be achieved by other means (particularly through the involvement of mentally competent patients).[14] (Taupitz and Frölich 1997, p. 913)

In this case, "justice has been done to the right to self-determination . . . if indications of solidarity for fellow human beings are taken seriously and these are granted as having legal significance for the question of the admissibility of research measures" (Taupitz and Frölich 1997, p. 913).

Consequently, respect for the right of self-determination means accepting the premise that every person has the right to decide, individually and according to his or her values and convictions, whether and how he or she wishes to act regarding his or her health (Beauchamp and Childress 1994). This corresponds to respect for personal attitudes, bodily integrity, and the private sphere of the patient as the constituent of his or her dignity. Respect for human dignity is expressed above all in interactions with the patient, more precisely in taking seriously his or her personal identity, the values and wishes that are known from the past. In the case of incompetent patients with dementia, this must all be traced and taken into consideration by his or her legal representative. It follows that research in medicine for which there is "no model which [could] be substituted for the human being . . . *also . . .* [constitutes] in every instance responsible, non-experimental interaction with the respective subject as an individual, which is 'to be taken seriously' " (Nagel 1996). The necessary factually oriented relationship with the patient must always be complemented by a value-oriented relationship. Only then is it possible to counter the objectivization of the research subject, conditioned by many scientific methods (not only with regard to the natural sciences) (Dörner 1996; Helmchen 1998b). The process by which the ethical dilemma is made conscious and by which measures are taken to ensure that the patient's dignity is respected acts to counter the mechanisms of dehumanization and secretiveness mentioned at the beginning of this chapter, and it also acts to counter the radicalization of any one principle.[15]

Subsequently, the Central Ethics Commission (Zentrale Ethikkommission 1997a) enumerated concrete protective criteria that minimize, in a defined fashion, the instrumentalization of the patient as well as possible risks for him or her:

- *"It must be impossible to carry out the research project with mentally competent patients."* This means that there are no alternative research strategies that can be used to answer the questions underlying this project (Fagot-Largeault 1996). If these questions can also be answered through research involving competent patients, this research project with incompetent patients is inadmissible. The following is an example of such a subject of inquiry, described elsewhere (Helmchen 1998a): An answer to the question of whether the pattern of psychopathological disorders and the speed of progression in later stages of dementia differ between young old patients (up to age 85 years) and very old patients (more than age 85 years) would be important in determining the extent to which dementia in old age represents merely accentuated aging or the expression of cerebral disease.
- *"The research project is expected to yield essential information about a disease, with regard to recognition, education, avoidance or treatment."* Accordingly, purely replicative "me too" research and research exclusively for the purpose of generating a hypothesis are indefensible. In making its assessment, the Ethics Commission should take into consideration the de-

gree to which research is needed. In the case of dementia, for example, re-search must be regarded as urgently needed, because the progression of dementia over a number of years means the continual suffering of the pa-tient and his or her next of kin, because the causes are still untreatable. In addition, the increasing occurrence of dementia means a growing burden on the public health care system, shown, not least of all, by the continuing discussion of the German Nursing Care Insurance Law (Bundesgesetzblatt I 1994 P. 1014, May 26, 1994). Furthermore, it is essential to note that any research involving mentally incompetent persons that benefits others ex-clusively is ethically indefensible according to the Declaration of Helsinki (1976); that is, all research interventions are excluded that have nothing to do with the illness of the patients involved.

♦ *"The risks involved in the research project are defensible in relation to the expected benefits."* In this form, the criterion can be applied only to re-search projects in which the patients involved can themselves reap bene-fit—if not immediately, then at least in the future course of their illness. In contrast, in research projects in which there is the promise of benefit not for the participants but only for other persons in the same age group or with the same disease, this criterion must be formulated more precisely: "At most, the research project is expected to involve minimal risks[16] or stress."

♦ *"The legal representative has given effective consent to the measures to be taken; this assumes that his or her knowledge of the person represented con-stitutes sufficient grounds to support the conclusion that the patient would consent to participating in the study."* In such situations, a living will made while the patient was mentally competent, or a power of attorney in medi-cal matters, could be helpful as an index of the patient's wishes. Here the guardian must not simply disregard the patient's concepts of solidarity with other patients simply because he or she has become mentally incom-petent.

♦ *"The patient involved does not demonstrate refusal by his or her behavior."* This means that the study must be terminated if the patient, and particu-larly the mentally incompetent patient, communicates that he or she wishes to end participation in the study.

♦ *"The appropriate Ethics Commission has adjudged the proposed research project affirmatively."* At least in controversial cases, the Ethics Commis-sion should submit written arguments with reference to the aforemen-tioned criteria, supporting its affirmative vote, and should recommend that a court decision be made, either directly or regarding the (emergency) appointment of a guardian.

The position paper contains concrete criteria for the determination of mental competence, because the incapacity to give informed consent is presupposed in dealing with mentally incompetent patients in research (Helmchen and Lauter 1995). Ethically, the question here is doing justice to the capacity of self-determination, thus to determine whether the person in this concrete case is capable of taking advantage of his or her right to self-determination.[17]

Criticisms

Finally, several more specific points of criticism in the public discussion should be mentioned, based on relevant recent German history:

- The medical motivation of research involving mentally incompetent persons stems from direct experience with patients (e.g., dementia patients, their relatives, and nursing personnel). Physicians want to be able to treat such illnesses more effectively than is currently possible and, therefore, in some cases, wish to include such mentally incompetent patients in research studies in which there is no other way to reach this goal. Indeed, incompetent patients are, in fact, more vulnerable because their illness (not the physician!) robs them of the capacity to exercise their own rights. For precisely this reason, physicians seek improvements in healing these illnesses or at least alleviating them to the extent that the patient regains the capacity to exercise his or her rights. Physicians do not wish—as is maintained by some critics—to make these patients "pliant" for purposes of research because they are so weak and vulnerable; on the contrary, physicians want to involve these patients in research under defined protective measures—such as the aforementioned—because the patients' illnesses are so severe and intractable that physicians are mandated to do something about them. This line of argument is also supported by the Physician's Code (Berufsordnung für Ärzte 1990), according to which the physician must also serve the population. However, this obligation is secondary and limited by the primary obligation of the physician to "serve the health of the individual human being" (Berufsordnung für Ärzte 1990, p. 1697).
- The individual and social desire for progress in treatment, particularly of severe illnesses, found expression in the 1964 Declaration of Helsinki (and its subsequent amendments), today generally recognized as the guideline for the ethical assessment of medical research and in which research involving mentally incompetent patients is recognized as ethically defen-

sible. This is in contradiction to the Nuremberg Code—a fact, however, that is explained by its historical context. The aim of this 1947 code was to condemn "research" involving nonconsenting, noninformed, duped human beings in National Socialist Germany; its authors did not mention research involving incompetent patients because they did not have such patients in mind, and the development of the need for therapeutic research including such patients could not have been foreseen, given the state of the art at that time (Meijers et al. 1995).

♦ Banning research involving mentally incompetent patients prevents the development of criteria and procedures through which to protect these patients, recognizing their particular vulnerability and maintaining ethical standards. Precisely such criteria and procedures appear to be necessary: on the one hand, the need is growing for research on severe illnesses, including those that can lead to mental incompetence (not only dementia but also cerebral traumas, strokes, cardiac breakdown, and forms of intoxication). In the United States in the 1980s, the widespread public opinion that tests with zidovudine (AZT) for AIDS were useful led physicians and patients to falsify criteria for inclusion in testing, revealing that measures intended to protect vulnerable individuals were circumvented when they did not appear to be an adequate solution to the problem at hand (Levine 1996). Another possible example could be that without criteria for determining mental competence, this state—defined very broadly with regard to clinical impressions—is assumed to be present or else the threshold used in explicitly examining it is set so high that the nonexistence of competence cannot be determined at all (Helmchen 1995). On the other hand, with the globalization of research and the worldwide application of research findings, there is the danger that the absolute exclusion of any kind of instrumentalization of human beings in one region could lead to uncontrolled and more extensive instrumentalization of human beings in another part of the world (Rössler 1996). In this case, the application in the first-mentioned regions of research findings from the latter would be ethically questionable.

♦ History has shown that the proclamation of ethical standards alone is not enough. It was mentioned earlier that the National Socialists committed their grave crimes despite state directives and that unethical research projects were also carried out after the Nuremberg Code was published. Continual debate is therefore urgently necessary regarding the increasingly broad spectrum of difficult ethical problems in medical research as well as in medical practice. The ethics commissions and public discussion represent steps in this direction. Although there appears to be no alternative to the institution of bodies of experts (Rössler 1996), it is nonetheless an important step forward that these experts carry into the public discussion their arguments in a comprehensible language and in a concentrated form summarizing the essential questions concerning position papers of the Scientific Advisory Board of the Federal Chamber of Physicians, the Central Ethics Commission, and professional organizations.

In light of modern German history, it is only understandable that discussion of research that exclusively benefits those other than the participating patients[18] and nontherapeutic research[19] with mentally incompetent patients has nourished fears of a medical science with inhuman characteristics. Because the risk of instrumentalization of human beings is inherent in this kind of research to a greater extent than in other kinds of medical intervention, such research deeply affects the fundamental human right to the recognition of personal dignity. Therefore, public discussion of this topic is necessary, not only because respect for human dignity is bound up with openness and the striving for understanding of others, but also because in an open society the understanding of opinions voiced is a precondition for those who have been invested with decision-making power in defining the parameters for such research. In this discussion, the philosophers should explicate the relationship between utilitarian and deontological ethics and the practical significance of this relationship, while the medical researchers have the task of defining individual and societal need for such research, of describing the concrete sequences—the complicated reality of benefit, risk, stress, and ethical justification of this research. Last but not least, part of the task is to articulate clearly the difficulties besetting our adherence to ethical principles in the complicated reality of medicine today, and that there are no simple solutions.

Conclusions

Medical research involving incompetent patients that is expected to yield only questionable or no individual benefit (and that is often wrongly equated with nontherapeutic research) remains a difficult and controversial problem (Helmchen 1998c). The structure of the inherent problems will be elucidated both in view of the experience of involvement of medical researchers in crimes against humanity in National Socialist Germany and in the context of our current knowledge about the mechanisms of becoming involved in such unethical behavior. The difficulty of the problem is reflected in the fact that such research is legally admissible in some countries, such as France and England, but is questionable or prohibited in other countries, such as Germany. From the standpoint of the physician, such research can only be justified if the need for it is defined according to specified criteria and the protective criteria are fulfilled, in particular to ensure that the instrumentalization of the patient that follows from his or her involvement in the research is held in check by observing respect for the patient's dignity, and furthermore to ensure that research does not involve more than minimal risks and negligible stress for the individual participant and that the patient's refusal to participate is accepted. A broad, international consensus exists with regard to these criteria (Dresser 1996; Keyserlingk et al. 1995; Law Commission 1993, 1995), but concepts and definitions must be developed further with regard to what constitutes benefits and risks—in particular, minimal risks.

Furthermore, there is a need for criteria, rules, and procedures to guide the weighing of benefits against risks and, not least of all, the weighing of individual benefit against social benefit. The following question must also be satisfactorily answered: Who is to do the weighing? But above all, it must be ensured by professional education that this process of checks and controls is effectively carried out in day-to-day medical-scientific life.

Endnotes

1. Thus, the murder of persons with mental illness was kept doubly secret despite propaganda that this action would bring relief from suffering and was necessary for economic reasons, to alleviate an intolerable burden on the economy. Externally it was carried out in great secret, and internally it was euphemistically termed *euthanasia.*

2. For example, the Tübingen psychiatrist and university "rector in SS uniform" H. Hoffman was not prepared to carry out his own preaching of "destruction of 'unworthy genes' by destroying life in the framework of the mass murder of the mentally ill" (Leonhardt et al. 1996, p. 951).

3. a) Klee (1997) described a Polish anthropologist who as a prisoner at Auschwitz went to work for the SS medical figure Mengele. As late as 1972, she considered his research findings to be very significant, and only in 1985 did she take an opposite position.

b) Finzen (1996) quoted from a 1935 essay by Eugen Bleuler describing his defense of euthanasia, albeit only to end individual suffering, as well as his simultaneous rejection of euthanasia for the purpose of alleviating the community burden.

c) In Holland, a majority of the population now supports voluntary euthanasia, which in Germany across the border brings to mind the horrible abuse of euthanasia by the National Socialists and which is viewed as a dangerous step on the road to criminality (Lauter and Meyer 1992).

d) The widespread eugenic movement of the first quarter of the twentieth century led, in the 1920s and 1930s in a considerable number of countries, to laws permitting forced sterilization, which in Sweden, despite the terrible experience of Germany, was practiced in the case of many thousands of human beings as late as 1976 (von Altenbeckum 1997). As early as 1907, the American state of Indiana introduced a law legalizing forced sterilization; by 1913 such laws were in force in 12 states. The U.S. Supreme Court confirmed the validity of these laws in 1927; in 1985 the laws were still in force in 19 states. In 1928 Denmark introduced a forced sterilization law, and the rest of Scandinavia followed suit in 1935 (Birley 1997).

Further-reaching questions follow from this: To what extent is the social consensus *(zeitgeist)* determined by the mere emotional reflexes (gut reactions) of a generation or an epoch, which in West Germany of the 1980s operated quite unconsciously on the self-evident understanding that the state is governed by law and that social welfare was secure, which a decade later had given way to a feeling of growing societal uncertainty? Thus, it can rightfully be conjectured that in the first decades after World War II, when memories of war and of the rule by violence with all its horrors were fresh, euthanasia was simply unthinkable; but that as another generation grew up and matured—on the one hand with the feeling of individual self-determination and the medical possibilities for alleviating suffering and on the other hand more and more generally experiencing the fragility and burden of old age—euthanasia has in the past two decades again become thinkable.

We live on shaky ground. The manifold ties anchoring us in society give us identity, stabilize us, and ensure that we do the right thing with regard to the norms of this society. At the same time, these ties are capable of allowing us as individuals to become "objectively" guilty if society develops in a negative, criminal direction, conditioned by the social consensus *(zeitgeist)*. In ancient tragedies, this "objective" process, of becoming guilty vis-à-vis principles personified or sanctioned by the gods, was depicted as the inevitability of fate, subjectively experienced as being not guilty. These "objective" principles—brought into existence by human beings but supposedly valid for human beings for all time and invariable—are human rights, codified by human rights conventions. But are they really invariable for all time, eternal? The development of jurisprudence points to opposite (even if it may not always lead to "good") conclusions.

4. For example, Martin Luther and Erasmus of Rotterdam were in favor of killing severely damaged newborn children out of pity (Dörner 1988; Walter 1948).

5. Compare Helmchen 1996.

6. For example, directly—after World War I and its consequences—and indirectly—as in the case of the considerable increase in the number of persons with conditions due to illness such as dementia or coma vigil. The latter in particular has recently led many to directly confront the problems discussed here, which are particularly evident at present, marked by increasing complaints regarding excessive health care costs.

7. Compare Helmchen and Vollmann 1999.

8. For example, Alvar and Gunnar Myrdal and the *Volksheim* concept in Sweden (von Altenbeckum 1997), or see Grotjahn 1912.

9. As has been shown by the advancement of scientists who were known worldwide before 1933, such as the psychiatrist Ernst Rüdin (Gottesman and Bertelsen 1996; Weber 1993) and the neuropathologist Julius Hallervorden (Daroff 1994; Peiffer 1997), or who were chairs of psychiatry departments after 1933, such as Carl Schneider in Heidelberg (Hohendorf et al. 1996) and Hermann Hoffmann in Tübingen (Leonhardt et al. 1996), or who were recognized as outstanding after 1945 as well, such as the neurologist Georges Schaltenbrand (Shevell and Evans 1994).

10. In reaction to the scandals in medical research at the end of the 19th century, the Prussian Royal Ministry for Cultural, Educational, and Medical Affairs issued clear guidelines on the *voluntary* participation of subjects in research studies. Again, in 1931, the German State Ministry of the Interior issued regulations governing *voluntary* participation and risk minimization in medical research, the unambiguous language of which is still unsurpassed (Vollmann and Winau 1996). These regulations obviously had no influence on subsequent catastrophic developments.

11. However, in this gray area, regulations are repeatedly overstepped, a fact that is often recognized only ex post facto. The desire to set procedures that are effective preventively is therefore understandable. On the other hand, one must keep in mind the dialectic of informed consent: the more precisely a life phenomenon is divided and subdivided, the more difficult it is to deal with it in practice according to regulations based on a rational analysis. Therefore, detailed regulations are effective only if they give rise to ongoing debate on the problem analyzed, particularly in medical education.

12. Nagel (1996) enumerated such cases, termed by him as dichotomies: 1) goals of an experiment (object)—respect for the subject; 2) freedom of decision making of the individual—society's obligation to care for the individual; and 3) the physician's responsibility vis-à-vis the individual patient—the physician's responsibility vis-à-vis society.

13. Is not the mandate of protection of life in health care institutions violated occasionally—but, because of the absolute quality of the mandate itself, secretively (Maisch 1997)? Is not consent occasionally assumed, to enable subject participation in a research study—but, because of the "bureaucratic" expense involved, not explicitly obtained?

14. This is excluded by the nature of some illnesses, such as dementia, that lead to mental incompetence. In other cases, such as legally regulated and obligatory vaccination, overwhelmingly mentally incompetent children—some of whom are exposed to a more than minimal risk—are subjected to preventive measures for the benefit of the community; the law governing epidemics provides for

measures to protect the community, according to which competent adults must also accept individual stress.

15. Above all, however, this also means setting and recognizing the threshold at which the principle (e.g., the right of self-determination) is affected in its essence or even called into question by virtue of its relationship to other principles (e.g., the welfare of the patient). Thus, conducting an objectively no-risk examination indicated by differential diagnosis (e.g., magnetic resonance imaging) in the case of a mentally incompetent dementia patient without going through the process of obtaining the consent of the guardian is ethically defensible if during the examination the patient can communicate with others and the examination is discontinued should he or she begin to have anxiety (i.e., if the patient is subjected to measures without risk that exclusively serve his or her own welfare and if his or her human dignity is respected). If the interest of research is also served by this examination, a guardian must exercise the right of the patient to self-determination.

16. With regard to the concept of minimal risks, the Central Ethics Commission (Zentrale Ethikkommission 1997a) wrote that it can be "determined only with difficulty but can be concretized by distinguishing among levels of risk and a list of examples. In any case, a distinction must be made between an objectifiable risk and subjective stress and/or complaints (e.g., a magnetic resonance image involves no objectifiable risks but can very well occasion subjective stress, leading to breaking off the examination). There is great individual variation and there are great differences among groups, in particular regarding subjective complaints. The Commission is of the opinion that one can speak of a 'minimal risk,' e.g., when a small amount of bodily fluid or tissue is removed in the course of diagnostic measures or surgical procedures that were necessary in any case and therefore involved no additional risk for the patient. Certain physical examinations (e.g., sonographs, transcutaneous tissue measurements, etc.) and certain psychological examinations (e.g., questionnaire interviews, tests, behavioral observations) fall into this group" (Zentrale Ethikkommission 1997a, p. B2195).

17. It is a question not of upholding the formal confirmation of consent but of doing justice to the patient's right of self-determination (e.g.,

not being too hasty to assume incompetence, in a case exclusively involving the health care of the patient; or not being too hasty to impute competence, in a case in which a research study is involved).

18. All research interventions for the sake of knowledge, transcending the individual patient, are at least also for the sake of others (i.e., including an attempt to heal).

19. Nontherapeutic (e.g., diagnostic) research can also bring direct potential individual benefit.

References

Beauchamp TL, Childress JF: Principles of Biomedical Ethics, 4th Edition. New York, Oxford University Press, 1994

Beecher KK: Ethics and clinical research. N Engl J Med 274:1354–1360, 1966

Berufsordnung für Ärzte. Amtsblatt für Berlin, September 14, 1990, p 1697

Birley JLT: Political abuse of psychiatry. Paper presented at the Geneva Initiative, Geneva, Switzerland, July 10, 1997

Burleigh M: Death and Deliverance: "Euthanasia" in Germany c. 1900–1945. Cambridge, England, Cambridge University Press, 1994

State v. Chabot, Supreme Court of the Netherlands, Criminal Chamber, 21 June 1994, No. 96.972. Nederlandse Jurisprudentie 1994, No. 665

Daroff RB: Schaltenbrand and Hallervorden. Neurology 44:201–202, 1994

Declaration of Helsinki. Recommendations guiding medical doctors in biomedical research involving human subjects. Med J Aust 1:206–207, 1976

Dörner K: Tödliches Mitleid. Zur Frage der Unerträglichkeit des Lebens, oder Die soziale Frage: Entstehung, Medizinisierung, NS-Lösung, heute, morgen. Gütersloh, Verlag Jakob von Hoddis, 1988

Dörner K: Wenn Ärzte nur das Beste wollen. Paper presented at the International Physicians for Prevention of Nuclear War Congress, Nuremberg, Germany, October 25–27, 1996

Dresser R: Mentally disabled research subjects: the enduring policy issues. JAMA 276:67–72, 1996

Erhardt H: Euthanasie und Vernichtung "lebensunwerten" Lebens. Stuttgart, Enke, 1965

Faden R (ed): The Human Radiation Experiments. New York, Oxford University Press, 1996

Fagot-Largeault A: National Report: France, in Informed Consent in Psychiatry. Edited by Koch HG, Reiter-Theil S, Helmchen H. Baden-Baden, Nomos, 1996, pp 67–96

Finzen A: Massenmord ohne Schuldgefühl. Bonn, Edition Das Narrenschiff im Psychiatrie-Verlag, 1996

Fuchs T, Lauter H: Der Fall Chabot: assistierter Suizid aus psychiatrischer Sicht. Nervenarzt 68:878–883, 1997

Griffiths J: Assisted suicide in the Netherlands: the Chabot case. Modern Law Review 58:232–248, 1995

Gottesman II, Bertelsen A: Legacy of German psychiatric genetics: hindsight is always 20/20. Am J Med Genet 67:317–322,1996

Groeben N: Wie war es möglich? Zur psychologischen Erklärbarkeit von Menschenversuchen im Dritten Reich, in Von der Heilkunde zur Massentötung—Medizin im Nationalsozialismus. Edited by Hohendorf G, Magull-Seltenreich A. Heidelberg, Hüthig, 1990, pp 203–228

Grotjahn A: Soziale Pathologie. Berlin, Springer, 1912

Hanuske-Abel HM: Not a slippery slope or sudden subversion: German medicine and National Socialism in 1933. BMJ 313:1453–1463, 1996

Helmchen H: Ethische Fragen in der Psychiatrie, in Psychiatrie der Gegenwart, 3rd Edition, Vol 2. Edited by Kisker KP, Lauter H, Meyer JE, et al. Berlin, Springer, 1996, pp 321–361

Helmchen H: Forschung mit nicht-einwilligungsfähigen Kranken. Berichte und Abhandlungen der Berlin-Brandenburgischen Akademie der Wissenschaften 5:9–30, 1998a

Helmchen H: Mutual patient-psychiatrist communication and the therapeutic contract. Compr Psychiatry 39:5–10, 1998b

Helmchen H: Research with patients incompetent to give informed consent. Current Opinion in Psychiatry 11:295–297, 1998c

Helmchen H, Lauter H (eds): Dürfen ärzte mit Demenzkranken forschen? Analyse des Problemfeldes Forschungsbedarf und Einwilligungsproblematik. Stuttgart, Thieme, 1995

Helmchen H, Vollmann J: Ethische Fragen in der Psychiatrie, in Psychiatrie der Gegenwart, 4th Edition, Vol 2. Edited by Helmchen H, Henn FA, Lauter H, et al. Berlin, Springer, 1999, pp 522–577

Hohendorf G, Roeicke V, Rotzoll M: Innovation und Vernichtung—Psychiatrische Forschung und "Euthanasie" an der Heidelberger Psychiatrischen Klinik 1939–1945. Nervenarzt 67:935–946, 1996

Hohendorf G, Roeicke V, Rotzoll M: Von der Ethik des wissenschaftlichen Zugriffs auf den Menschen: die Verknüpfung von psychiatrischer Forschung und "Euthanasie" im Nationalsozialismus und einige Implikationen für die heutige Diskussion in der medizinischen Ethik. Beiträge zur NS-Gesundheits- und Sozialpolitik 13:81–106, 1997

Keyserlingk EW, Glass K, Kogan S, et al: Proposed guidelines for the participation of persons with dementia as research subjects. Perspect Biol Med 38:319–361, 1995

Klee E: Auschwitz, die NS-Medizin und ihre Opfer. Frankfurt, Fischer, 1997

Lauter H, Meyer JE: Die neue Euthanasie—Diskussion aus psychiatrischer Sicht. Fortschr Neurol Psychiatr 60:441–448, 1992

Law Commission: Mentally Incapacitated Adults and Decision Making: Medical Treatment and Research (Consultation Paper 129). London, Her Majesty's Stationery Office, 1993

Law Commission: Mental Incapacity (HC Paper 189). London, Her Majesty's Stationery Office, 1995

Leonhardt L, Foerster K: Hermann F. Hoffmann (1891–1844)—die Tübinger Psychiatrie auf dem Weg in den Nationalsozialismus. Nervenarzt 67:947–952, 1996

Levine RJ: Proposed regulations for research involving those institutionalized as mentally infirm: a consideration of their relevance. Institutional Review Board: A Review of Human Subjects Research (Hastings Center) 18:1–5, 1996

Maisch H: Patiententötungen—dem Sterben nachgeholfen. Munich, Kindler, 1997

Meijers LCM, de Boer J, Kommission medizinisch Experimente mit Einwilligungsunfähigen: Medizinisch wissenschaftliche Untersuchungen mit Einwilligungsunfähigen [Medical Experiments With Incapacitated Persons]. Report to the Ministry for Health, Welfare and Sport and the Ministry of Justice, The Hague, May 16, 1995

Meyer-Lindenberg J: The Holocaust and German psychiatry. Br J Psychiatry 159:7–12, 1991

Mitscherlich A, Mielke F: Das Diktat der Menschenverachtung. Heidelberg, Schneider, 1947

Mitscherlich A, Mielke F: Medizin ohne Menschlichkeit. Dokumente des Nürnberger Ärzteprozesses. Frankfurt, Fischer, 1960

Nagel E: Historische Erfahrungen und ärztliches Handeln: ethische Verpflichtungen bei Therapie und Forschung am Menschen. Paper presented at the 99th German Physicians Congress, Köln, Germany, June 5, 1996

Nursing Care Insurance Law (Pflege-Versicherungsgesetz). Bundesgesetzblatt I 1994 P. 1014-1073, 26 May 1994

Peiffer J: Hirnforschung im Zwielicht: Beispiele verführbarer Wissenschaft aus der Zeit des Nationalsozialismus; Hallervorden J, Scherer H-J, Ostertag B (Abhandlungen zur Geschichte der Medizin und der Naturwissenschaften, issue 79). Husum, Matthiesen, 1997

Rössler D: Zur Diskussion über die Bioethik-Konvention. Ethik in der Medizin 8:167–172, 1996

Schmidt G: Selektion in der Heilanstalt 1939–1945. Stuttgart, Evangelisches Verlagswerk, 1965

Shevell MI, Evans BK: The "Schaltenbrand experiment," Würzburg 1941: scientific, historical and ethical perspectives. Neurology 44:350–356, 1994

Taupitz J, Fröhlich U: Medizinische Forschung mit nicht-einwilligungsfähigen Personen. Versicherungs Recht 22:911–918, 1977

Vollmann J, Winau R: Informed consent in human experimentation before the Nuremberg Code. BMJ 313:1445–1448, 1996 von Altenbeckum J: "Nazismus mit umgekehrtem Gedankengang" in Schweden. Frankfurter Allgemeine Zeitung, September 2, 1997

Walter F: Die Euthanasie und die Heiligkeit des Lebens: die Lebensvernichtung im Dienste der Medizin und Eugenik nach christlicher und monistischer Ethik. Munich, Max Hueber, 1948

Weber MM: Ernst Rüdin: eine kritische Biographie. Berlin, Springer, 1993

Weindling R: Weimar eugenics: the Kaiser Wilhelm Institute for Anthropology, Human Heredity and Eugenics in social context. Annals of Science 42:303–318, 1985

Zentrale Ethikkommission: Stellungnahme. Deutches Ärzteblatt 94:B2194–B2196, 1997a

Zentrale Ethikkommission: Zum Schutz nicht-einwilligungsfähiger Personen in der medizinischen Forschung. Deutches Ärzteblatt 94:A1911–A1912, 1997b

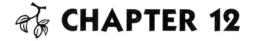

CHAPTER 12

Informed Consent

A Historical and Medical Perspective

Prof. Dr. Dr. Jochen Vollmann

Today, informed consent of patients is a standard and basic ethical principle. Before any medical intervention, the patient or the person involved should explicitly express his or her consent. For consent to be given, the doctor must inform the patient of the objective, the benefit, and the risks of the intervention and must also inform the patient of any possible alternative interventions. To be able to use this information in autonomous decision making, the patient must have understood the information and must be capable of giving free consent (i.e., must be able to make a decision without outside pressure, coercion, or manipulation). A patient able to give consent is able to apply the understood information to his or her own personal situation, to identify the consequences of his or her decision through rational and sequential thought, and to weigh the advantages against the disadvantages of his or her choice. The patient should furthermore have a quasi-realistic insight into his or her personal situation (illness), acknowledge the diagnostic or therapeutic possibilities, and reach a decision that he or she can communicate (Appelbaum and Grisso 1995). Informed consent, there-

This chapter is based on Vollmann J: "Das Informed-Consent-Konzept als Politikum in der Medizin. Patientenaufklärung und Einwilligung aus historischer und medizinethischer Perspektive," in *Angewandte Ethik als Politikum*. Edited by Kettner M. Frankfurt, Suhrkamp, 2000, pp. 253–279.

167

fore, involves being given information, understanding the information, being able to consent, and having free choice (Faden and Beauchamp 1986; Vollmann 1996). Through informed consent, the attempt is made to ensure that patients are not abused as objects of modern medicine and that they are acknowledged as independent, responsible persons whose rights and private space must be respected.

From a legal point of view, informing the patient is a prerequisite for a patient's consent to a line of management, which would otherwise have been considered a forbidden challenge of the integrity of a human being—in legal terms a physical injury. On the basis of these legal considerations, informing the patient has gained considerable importance in clinical practice. In the absence of such adequate information, a physician would bear the legal responsibility of a professional mistake should the patient decide to complain in court. Therefore, formal, legally sound documentation of the patient's consent has been considered more and more important in recent years.

Historical Development

This concept of informed consent in medicine tends to be discussed in the literature of bioethics as if it were a development of the second half of the twentieth century (Faden and Beauchamp 1986; Levine 1986; Veatch 1995). In traditional medical ethics—for example, in the Hippocratic Oath—self-determination and freedom of choice of patients in a medical context was hardly addressed; rather, the focus was on virtuous behavior, beneficence toward the patient, and protection from nonmaleficence.

These medical ethics were unquestioningly valid until the second half of the twentieth century. Even at the time of the European Renaissance nothing seemed to have changed in the reality of the patronizing attitude of members of the medical profession. The philosophical aspect of that enlightenment, however, spilled over into medicine and there was criticism of the minimal attention given to some enlightened and reasonable arguments on the part of the patient.[1] There was, however, hardly any reference to the physician's informing the patient about the realities of his or her illness, the suggested management, or the patient's consent as a sign of respect or consideration of the patient's autonomy. The certificate of medical practice, valid until today and created by the World Medical Association in 1948, is similar to the Hippocratic Oath in ignoring the physician's commitment to informed consent (Bundesärztekammer 1990, 1994).[2]

Whereas the right to the final assessment regarding a patient's well-being was attributed to the doctor in classical medical ethics, Veatch (1995) stated that a patient's consent was given ethical value in the second half of the twentieth century. However, a more detailed examination of the historical development of informed consent in the doctor-patient relationship reveals a more complex process that requires a more analytical approach for understanding. It is methodologically problematic to isolate the contemporary concept of informed consent from its social and historical origins in other historical epochs and circumstances.

It is necessary, therefore, to define more accurate criteria that should be satisfied in the education and consent of patients in earlier historical epochs. In doing so, one should not, on the one hand, set a very high standard to avoid a nonreflective mechanical transfer of modern concepts onto earlier historical times and thereby lose trace of the historical foundations of the concepts of education and consent. On the other hand, one would need to formulate concretely defined criteria for the process of informing the patient and obtaining consent from the patient and his or her relatives to be able to do justice to the concept. Faden and Beauchamp (1986) suggested the following criteria for the description and interpretation of patient's consent in the history of medicine:

1. The patient or research subject should agree to the intervention on the basis of comprehensive information received.
2. Consent should not be obtained by coercion.
3. Consent should entail a conscious permission for a concrete intervention (i.e., the patient or research subject should consent explicitly and there should be no room for misunderstanding).

A further problem in the search for the historical roots of informed consent in medicine lies in the limitation of sources. Available objective information is frequently not enough to apply the above mentioned criteria. There is therefore great space for interpretation (Faden and Beauchamp 1986). For example, the earlier restricted spectrum of anesthetic possibilities meant that a surgical intervention could not be carried out without the patient's cooperation. This cooperation alone, however, cannot be taken to indicate fulfillment of the first of the criteria just listed. Furthermore, a differentiation should be made between informed consent on the one hand and truthfulness at the sick bed on the other, a subject of long historical discussion (Lederer 1995).[3] Even when a doctor informs the patient of the diagnosis and prognosis of the condition, it does not follow that the patient has contributed his or her choice to the line of management, because the doctor, irrespective of the information he or she conveys, can still decide on the management alone, without having to ask for the patient's consent (criteria 1 and 3). It is even more difficult to assess the impact of the institution in the case of hospitalized mentally ill or disabled persons (criterion 2), when there is rarely any information regarding the content of the necessary patient education. Frequently, one can draw only on doctors' diaries, medical regulations or oaths, professional literature, newspaper clippings, and fiction—hardly directly on patients' stories—to learn about the practice of patient education at that time. Furthermore, one must be certain whether these historical sources (e.g., medical codes of practice and regulations) were the true reflection of the management practice or merely fulfilled the role of idealistic guidelines, a tool for political consensus or a tool of professional self-protection (Faden and Beauchamp 1986).

In American literature on bioethics, the year of the birth of informed consent is frequently cited as being 1957, when informed consent became case law through a ruling by the U.S. Supreme Court. More recent historical research, however, indicates an earlier existence of a medico-ethical debate within the medical profession, the legal profession, and political circles and publicly, regarding what the doctor was permitted to do with and without the patient's consent. Already used in those debates, taking place toward the end of the nineteenth century, were terms such as *truth, information, consent,* and collaboration in the doctor-patient relationship, especially in the field of clinical research. The American medical historian Susan Lederer (1995) showed that since before the Second World War, there had been critical ethical discussions regarding medical therapeutic trials within the medical profession as well as in the public media. Modern therapeutic research involving humans and ethical regulation through the medical profession itself as well as through state regulations had already begun before the frequently quoted Nuremberg Code (1947). Between 1890 and 1940, there was discussion in medical professional journals and at medical congresses about "unethically" conducted therapeutic and nontherapeutic research, discussion that was frequently accompanied and resolved by open criticism (Lederer 1995).[4] Lederer's research results showed that the hitherto predominant image of medicine as rich in scientific knowledge but also ethically uncontrolled and involving experimentation on human beings had already lost credibility and foundation before World War II. The abuse of research subjects and patients in medical research and the critical discussions within the medical profession and among the public regarding that abuse were important triggers for regulations and guidelines governing the education and obtaining of consent of patients or research subjects.

In 1874, the American Medical Association resolved to condemn a concrete case of unethical medical experimentation involving a patient with an incurable condition[5] and concluded that harming patients in the name of science was unacceptable in American medicine because it violates the cardinal medical principle of avoiding harming the patient (Lederer 1995). In this resolution, the condemnation relates not to the lack of patient education and consent but rather to the violation of the nonmaleficence principle. Earlier on, the case had been reported in a distinguished medical journal with no objection by the publishers. The case attracted the attention of the American Medical Association only after heavy criticism was received from British doctors who had learned about the case from the medical journal. It would be correct to interpret the exceptionally sharp and open condemnation of the American Medical Association as an international as well as a national harm-restricting measure.

In 1891, the Academy of Medicine in France described a medical research project on the transmissibility of cancer[6] as "criminal" and refused to permit scientific discussion of it. In July 1891, the Prussian Royal Ministry for Cultural, Educational, and Medical Affairs carried out an official investigation of the clinical research of surgeons Eugen Hahn and Ernst von Bergmann, who had undertaken similar operations, albeit with a palliative intention.[7] In that case, reference was made to the patients' desperate need for any operation, even those expected to do no good. Despite that need, however, they did not consent to participate in the experiment. The arguments in those cases were based on the principle of nonmaleficence (Lederer 1995).

In 1907, the prominent American clinician William Osler made a statement at the Congress of American Physicians and Surgeons indicating his view that the limits of human experiments are well defined and clear. Although experimentation on humans cannot be avoided in the field of clinical research, it is only allowed after extensive and detailed animal experimentation. Only after animal experimentation has resulted in the highest possible safety margin is the physician allowed, after full patient consent, to try the new therapy on humans. Osler stated that physicians do not have the right to use their trusting patients as experimental subjects if the patients will not directly benefit from the experiments. On the other hand, the physician has other ethical responsibilities when he or she carries out nontherapeutic medical experiments on healthy subjects. As long as the research subject is informed of the full implications of the circumstances surrounding the experiment and expresses willingness to participate in the experiment, these experiments not only are permitted but also should be praised, because—despite some occasional regrettable incidents—they constitute invaluable contributions to the advancement of medical research.

Osler's position in 1907 was remarkable. First, it introduced the condition of prior animal experimentation, a condition that would be endorsed in the Nuremberg Code in 1947, as well as in the Declaration of Helsinki of the World Medical Association (Bundesärztekammer 1991), and that is still relevant today. Second, his differentiation between therapeutic research (research involving some potential benefit for the patient) and nontherapeutic research (referred to by Osler as "medical experiment") is still used, with different ethical regulations applied to each of them. Furthermore, Osler's position means that the issue of informed consent was introduced into the medical debate of the American medical profession as early as the beginning of the twentieth century.

In response to the multiple, partially questionable experiments involving tuberculin injections in humans, the Prussian Ministry of the Interior in Germany issued a decree on February 28, 1891, that "the use of Dr. Koch's substance on tuberculous prisoners without their consent should be forbidden" (quoted in Vollmann and Winau 1996). It should be highlighted here that reference is made to ill prisoners (i.e., patients whose freedom and freedom of choice are limited because of imprisonment). Despite, or rather because of, this compulsory detention, the Ministry decided that tuberculin, an experimental therapeutic agent at that time, could not be tried on those patients against their will. We cannot, however, deduce a position vis-à-vis patients' active expression of will, not to mention informed consent (Lederer 1995).[8]

The central relevance of patient consent as a legitimizing condition for medical intervention is also highlighted in the German court ruling on May 31, 1894 (Reichsgericht 1894).[9] Surgical intervention is an injury to the body undertaken by surgeons with the purpose of healing. From a rights perspective, it is patient consent and not the physicians' professional right to the decision that allows for such intervention. The Royal Court expressed its position that the doctor can take action in the interest of the patient without the autonomous consent of the respective patient (or his or her representative).

To draw on one's personal conviction or the judgement of professional colleagues that a certain clever and accurate intervention would positively influence the physical or psychic well-being of a patient and to believe that one is better able to identify the real interests of a person than the person him or herself does not grant one the right, based on one's assessment, to encroach on the rights of that person, to violate his or her space and use him or her as an object of a well-motivated healing experiment. The absurdity of such a position becomes evident when we consider that the herein claimed "right," even if it is based on a reasonable cause, would consequently lead to raising one's subjective estimation, one's subjective belief in one's capacity and meticulousness to act in the welfare of the other, to the level of a right building, right granting and right determining factor. (Reichsgericht 1894 [RGSt 25, 375])

The individual patient's consent is a determining factor in the doctor-patient relationship and the decision-making process regarding any management intervention. The patient is at any time entitled to object to a therapeutic process or the use of any single therapeutic method used on him or her (Elkeles 1989; Reichsgericht 1894). This statement of rights was adopted by the Federal Supreme Court (Bundesgerichtshof in Strafsachen 11, 112; 16, 309), although the negative effect of a medical intervention on the integrity of the human body and the role of the patient's consent have been contested since the nineteenth century (Held 1990).

In European and American medical history, there are further examples of ethical debates on human experimentation (Faden and Beauchamp 1986; Lederer 1995). In that regard, I will discuss two important European regulations that, despite their relevance to modern medical ethics, have hardly been mentioned (Sass 1983).

Prussian Decree
of 1900

The instruction issued by the Prussian Royal Ministry for Cultural, Educational, and Medical Affairs on December 9, 1900, addressed to owners of clinics, polyclinics, and any forms of institutions for patients, is the oldest known state regulation. It required "objective provision of information" and "doubtless consent" with regard to nontherapeutic experiments on humans (Vollmann and Winau 1996, p. 410). The production of this very early document on informed consent was not an initiative of the medical profession or a research institution. Rather, it was the outcome of public criticism, expressed by the political media and parliament, of the abuse of human beings in scientific experiments[10] (Elkeles 1985; Tashiro 1991). Thus, informed consent was not a product of the medical profession but a legal model, in which, as early as 1900, the attempt was made to conceptualize the notions of informing the patient and patient consent as acclaimed legal rights of the patient. The attribution of responsibility was hierarchical according to Prussian legislation. The director of any patient institution had to bear full and exclusive responsibility for all clinical research carried out on human beings within his or her sector. It therefore followed that only the doctor (or doctors) in charge was authorized to carry out human research. Furthermore, special protection was granted to minors and patients who were not completely competent— the latter being especially relevant for psychiatry—and documentation of written consent was compulsory.

Guidelines for New Therapies and Scientific Experiments on Humans

In the 1930s, the State Minister of the Interior issued a circular indicating that his office would for the first time regulate all forms of informed consent for each form of clinical research that involved humans (Sass 1983). The trigger of this political process, which eventually produced the state guidelines, was the catastrophe induced by the Lübeck BCG (bacillus Calmette-Guerin) vaccine, which involved the death of 68 people, most of whom were children. In the court trial that followed, it was ruled that vaccine trials were to be managed strictly as medical experiments, which require the informed consent of the parents of children to be vaccinated. The state guidelines went into force in February 1931 and were relevant for all practicing doctors in the Weimar Republic.

In the guidelines, it was acknowledged that medical science and therapy cannot progress without scientific research involving human beings. It followed from this that the doctor had not only a right to carry out such research but also a duty toward and major responsibility for the life and health of every single research subject. At the same time, along the lines of Osler's position in 1907, a differentiation was made between therapeutic experiments (trials of new therapies) and nontherapeutic experiments (scientific experiments), preceded by introductory animal experimentation and a harm-benefit assessment. Scientific experiments had to meet stricter criteria than did therapeutic experiments. Both had to meet strict professional and scientific criteria according to the "rules of the medical art and science," undergo risk-benefit analysis, and involve informed consent. There was mention of "provision of information, inclusive of purpose," and an explanation of the consequences of consent that is detailed and concrete, leaving "no space for misunderstanding" (quoted in Sass 1983, pp. 99–111).

Whereas the consent component was standardized, there was some room for interpretation in the component of providing information, especially as far as the purpose of the experiment is concerned. The terms *informing* and *instructing* suggest a paternalistic doctor-patient relationship, in which the doctor is the expert, privileged because of a superior level of knowledge, and a moral authority in instructing. In cases in which the instructions relate to the objective of the study, one should critically question whether the instructions are primarily patient oriented (i.e., whether they include information about alternative therapies). On the other hand, patients were given room for independent decision making in the aspect of consent. Furthermore, doctors had to provide written documentation of the research protocol and the process by which they obtained the informed consent.

Minors received special protection. Consideration was given to protecting patients and research subjects from exposure in scientific publications. Experiments that involved microorganisms were assessed in light of the danger of infection of the population. Guidelines were sensitive to the limitations imposed by social and institutional contexts in which the research was taking place; in this respect, these guidelines extended beyond the Nuremberg Code as well as the Declaration of Helsinki. Taking advantage of social disadvantage for the sake of carrying out therapeutic research, not to mention nontherapeutic research, was condemned.[11]

The introduction of scientific research methodology into clinical medicine—especially methodology that derived from physiology, bacteriology, and immunology—led to an increase in hospital-based experimental research involving patients. Within this new structure of power and responsibility, the individual responsibility of the treating physician vis-à-vis his or her patient was complemented by that of the chief physician, who was responsible for all clinical human research undertaken in the institution. This hierarchical structure of ethical responsibility in clinical research, already present in the Prussian ordinance, is contradictory to structures in modern international developments, in which ethical responsibility is not regulated within the hierarchy of the clinic but is given to the independent researcher, who is advised by interdisciplinary, independent ethics committees.[12]

Finally, the 1931 guidelines called for medical curricula to incorporate a mention of the ethical duties of the researching doctor. Nonetheless, these guidelines have hardly been considered in bioethical discussions of informed consent.

The 1931 guidelines, which were still in force during the Third Reich, could not prevent the horrible human research carried out by German doctors in concentration camps. It is a frightening coincidence that the country that very early in history had produced state guidelines for clinical research involving humans would, under Nazi rule, witness such inhumane experimentation on human beings.

Patient Instruction and Consent in Clinical Human Research

The existence of the guidelines just discussed should not allow us, however, to draw conclusions regarding the daily practice of patient instruction and consent. The few documents on real medical research involving human beings reflect a completely different picture. For example, Neisser, toward the end of the nineteenth century, defended himself against the reproach that he had experimented on patients without informing them nor obtaining their consent. He not only denied the danger and risks involved in his experiment, which necessarily would have called for informed consent; but basically also rejected the concept altogether. He did not inform his female patients nor request their consent because, in his words,

> from a moral standpoint, I did not give any weight to their consent and I would never do. If I was concerned with a formal coverage of my work, I would have definitely got their consent, because there is nothing easier than to use friendly conversation in order to convince substance-ignorant subjects to provide you with any desired consent, especially if it has to do with such harmless daily practice like an injection. I would only speak of a consent if the matter had to do with people who are capable on the basis of their own knowledge and observation to fully understand the potentially possible risks. (quoted in Tashiro 1991, p. 93)

This statement clearly reveals what little value was given by medical researchers to patients' choice. Because patients did not possess any medical knowledge, it was assumed that they had no capacity to consent (Kuttig 1993).

This paternalistic representation of the patient could be found even among doctors who were critical of the research practice of their times and who generally approved of informing their patients and obtaining their consent. The Berlin-based psychiatrist Albert Moll (1902), for example, in his book on medical ethics, expressed his belief that all mentally ill patients are unable to consent and that consent should be obtained from relatives.

It is worrying to consider how such beliefs might have affected the attitude of psychiatrists treating patients with so-called war neurosis. Because of the life-threatening nature of some psychiatric treatments,[13] the Ministry of War decreed, on December 6, 1915, that in the case of very dangerous treatment methods, the doctor should obtain the soldier's consent (Riedesser and Verderber 1985). Kehrer (1917), a psychiatrist from Freiburg, objected to that:

In relation to treatment, there still remains the issue of the patient's freedom of choice of the treatment method to be used. Fortunately, when it comes to this matter, we are as protected as we are determined. The Ministry of War has decided that the patient's consent is only needed in cases of major intervention, where there is need for any form of narcotic, inclusive of chlorethyl inhalation. Still there remains the question whether the patient has to consent to the method used. I cannot, even on the basis of medical grounds, identify any rationale that justifies the consent of the patient to the choice of method. I rather believe that it would be best for the psychic well-being of the soldier not to exclude the medical cure, which should in all conditions be performed by a medical superior, from the principle of absolute obedience. (p. 18)

This statement is a demonstration of a psychiatrist's attributing less importance to a patient's consent to life-threatening interventions than was attributed by the Ministry of War during World War I.

Hall (1996) analyzed 380 reports on psychiatric clinical drug trials published in German-speaking professional journals between 1844 and 1952 and found only 12 pieces of research in which the informed consent of the patients or their relatives was mentioned. These trials involved the testing of electroconvulsive, fever, and malaria therapy on hospitalized patients.

In three of those studies, the idea of patient consent was "naturally" rejected, so that subjectivity issues would not influence test results. In one study, even psychiatrically healthy controls were not informed of the expected effects and side effects of the drug. With regard to fever therapy, the consent of research subjects or their relatives was obtained. However, the investigators left open the decision about whether such consent was at all necessary. Consent was rarely not given. However, the doctors still believed that the procedure led to unnecessary discomfort for the relevant subjects. A country psychiatric hospital developed a consent form that was meant to inform subjects of the procedures of the planned insulin therapy program. The form stated: "[Because] the treatment is invasive and can—albeit in rare cases—induce a threat to life, we would like to inform you of our intentions. Should you wish to discuss the issue, our doctor will be happy to help. If we do not hear from you within 8 days, we shall assume that you have consented" (quoted in Hall 1996). Another psychiatrist reported: "In many cases of written consent to treatment by relatives, we come across difficulties and frequently stubborn rejection. However, in cases where information is given verbally by the doctor, we are hardly ever denied consent. It is, therefore, recommended, whenever possible, to obtain a verbal consent for insulin therapy from the patients" (quoted in Hall 1996). From the available literature, it is not clear whether the conversation between doctor and relative was used for the purpose of informed consent or for manipulation of the relative into consent. Formulations and quotes in scientific publications tend to indicate a "teaching" attitude and a one-sided instructing process geared toward the interest of the doctor, with less importance placed on patient self-determination and choice.

Historical Interpretation

The American historian Martin S. Pernick demonstrated in his works on the history of medicine in the nineteenth century that being truthful to the patient and making an effort to obtain patient consent were part and parcel of the medical tradition at that time. This attitude was based on the theory that respect for informing the patient and patient autonomy had a positive impact on treatment outcome and thus contributed to the well-being of the patient. True, Pernick admitted that the nineteenth-century meaning of and motives behind obtaining informed consent were different from modern meaning and motives; the nineteenth-century concept of informed consent was, because of the different social context, not rights oriented but rather was based on the traditional principle of beneficence. Despite different social contexts and rationalization strategies, Pernick believed that there existed in the nineteenth century a medical practice that was concerned with establishing meaningful consent practices (Pernick 1982). His arguments were later supported in a wide legal discussion and later in court. Katz (1984) acknowledged this support but at the same time indicated that the judicial developments reflected little of the reality of the doctor-patient relationship. Frequently a doctor would fail to convey some information to the patient in order to be able to obtain the patient's consent and ensure the patient's cooperation in treatment. In this case, the issue is not one of relevant consent, because the patient is not granted the right of choice (Katz 1984).

It seems that Pernick and others tend to agree that patients in the nineteenth century were informed of the medical interventions and that in most cases they freely consented to undergo those interventions. Whether meaningful consent was obtained remains controversial. Furthermore, the social historical context and the impact of law and court decisions on the doctor-patient relationship were differently interpreted. For further discussion, the different definitions of consent become of utmost importance. In Pernick's concept of consent, meaningful consent is possible on the basis of information given, even if autonomy is absent and the beneficence principle is maintained. Faden and Beauchamp (1986) agreed with the historical and social analysis of the doctor-patient relationship and proceeded to use the exact meaning of consent in their work, that meaning being that a patient or research subject is outspoken and equally entitled to choose and consent.

Despite this difference in historical interpretation of informed consent, the aforementioned authors agreed that toward the end of World War II, at the latest, the concept of education and autonomous consent as a right was introduced into medical ethics (Moll 1902).[14]

The Nuremberg Code

In the context of the Nuremberg trials of 1945–1946, 20 doctors and 3 administrative employees were accused of carrying out human experiments in Nazi concentration camps that violated the human rights of people and were frequently fatal (Annas and Grodin 1992; Mitscherlich and Mielke 1947, 1949). What we refer to today as the Nuremberg Code is a component of the court judgment of August 19, 1947, in *United States v. Karl Brandt et al.* Brandt was involved in medical experimentation during the Second World War (Jäckel 1996).[15]

The judges argued on the basis of natural rights and referred to universally relevant moral, ethical, and rights principles[16] and thereby established that patients' rights in clinical research are universal and inalienable. The voluntary consent of a human being as well as sufficient knowledge and comprehension are, by virtue of right, preconditions for carrying out experiments on human beings. On the one hand, information and consent became rights-related preconditions of medical research involving humans. They became an acclaimed right of patients or their relatives and were meant to protect them from abuse. American judges consequently drew on the medical participation in Nazi experiments and replaced the medical beneficence principle with the principle of patient autonomy. On the other hand, the duty to carefully carry out research and assume the responsibility for that research remains solely that of the doctor. Concrete statements, similar to those in the German guidelines of 1931, are made in that context: Human experiments are allowed only after animal experiments have been carried out and must have as their aim fruitful results that positively affect the well-being of humankind and that cannot be obtained by other methods. The experiments should avoid all unnecessary suffering or harm; they cannot be carried out if death or invalidity are possible consequences. The risk should by no means outweigh the humanitarian relevance of the research outcome, and the safety of the research subject is top priority during the research. The research subject has the right to interrupt the research at any time, and researchers have the duty to terminate the research if major harm could be inflicted on the research subject.

The Nuremberg Code expanded the beneficence principle with the patient's right to autonomous informed freedom of choice. In accordance with this code, the doctor is obliged to prepare a responsible, solid research plan inclusive of a risk-benefit analysis. The patient should then be requested to give autonomous and informed consent to participate in the experiment, for which the doctor is claiming full responsibility. This new concept of informed consent, inclusive of autonomy, beneficence, and entitlement principles, served in following years as a model for various guidelines (Faden and Beauchamp 1986). The sustained impact of the Nuremberg Code, in contrast to all earlier guidelines, was evident in the United States in the 1950s and early 1960s, when the new informed consent concept was translated into a component of public policy. Whereas there were only 9 American publications dealing with issues of consent between 1930 and 1956, the number of publications on informed consent increased exponentially between 1960 and 1980, with more than 1,000 papers published in 1980 alone (Kaufmann 1983).

Faden and Beauchamp (1986) linked those developments with complex social developments. The modern concept of informed consent developed outside medicine, as a legal concept that rapidly entered American case law.[17] With the first case, in 1957, the modern concept of informed consent entered law in the United States, and from then on informed consent received great consideration in the medical community. The simultaneous development of interdisciplinary bioethics in the United States allowed the incorporation of a medical perspective in the rights perspective of the informed consent principle. Sociopolitical developments such as the civil rights movement and the consumer rights movement led to greater autonomy, individualism, and political awareness, which expressed themselves in the medical field through stronger patient rights.[18] Furthermore, unethical medical experiments carried out by American doctors, especially during the Second World War and the Cold War years, were made public and led to a critical public attitude toward medical experimentation (Charles R. McCarthy, "Research Ethics: Background and Contemporary Problems," Kennedy Institute of Ethics, Georgetown University, Washington, DC, 1994).

The Declaration of
Helsinki (1989 Version)

In accordance with the Nuremberg Code, the 1989 version of the Declaration of Helsinki (originally issued by the World Medical Association in 1964) included recommendations to doctors worldwide who were involved in biomedical research. In addition to the previously mentioned basic principles of the Nuremberg Code, the declaration requires the establishment of ethics committees for the supervision of research and includes more detailed regulations for the process of informed consent. "Not fully competent" research subjects should have legal representatives who should ensure that the research protocol meets the necessary ethical criteria. As in the guidelines of 1931, there is differentiation between therapeutic research (clinical experiments) and nontherapeutic research involving humans. For the latter, research subjects are defined as healthy individuals or patients whose condition is not related to the objective of the research.

Although the World Medical Association recommended the informed consent model, it introduced an exceptional regulation regarding therapeutic research involving humans: "If the doctor estimates that it is absolutely necessary to bypass the informed consent of the patient, then the reasons for this exception should be clearly defined in the independent components of the research protocol" (Bundesärztekammer 1991). Specialists in medical ethics strongly criticized this regulation and expressed their concern that the established right of the patient to unconstrained informed consent might again be bypassed in favor of medical paternalistic beneficence. This toning-down tendency can also be found in the international ethical guidelines for biomedical human research issued by the Council for International Organizations of Medical Sciences and the World Health Organization in 1993 (Annas 1995). The majority of the medical profession would accept the Declaration of Helsinki as a significant milestone in the effort to reach consensus on the principle of informed consent in human research (Faden and Beauchamp 1986). Many national guidelines have oriented themselves according to the declaration (e.g., the statement of the U.S. Food and Drug Administration of 1981 [Levine 1986] and the statement of the National Commission for the Protection of Human Subjects of Biomedical and Behavioral Research [Levine 1986]). In Germany, relevant regulations include the drug law (Deutsche Arzneimittelgesetz [AMG]; Sander 1993) and the professional regulations for physicians (Bundesärztekammer 1990, 1994).

Summary

In traditional medical ethics, as expressed in the Hippocratic Oath, the virtuous attitude of the doctor toward the well-being of his or her patients is placed at the forefront. In this case, however, well-being and harm are unilaterally considered from the professional point of view of the doctor. It remains to be defined how a treating doctor could act for the well-being of his or her individual patient without asking the patient about his or her values and wishes. The ethical debate on giving accurate information to the patient and patient consent in relation to medical human experiments can be traced to no earlier than the nineteenth century.

Difficult and frequently fatal consequences of medical human research have led to court cases and open controversy both within the medical profession and among the public. These legal and political arguments led to the placement of greater value on patient consent in modern scientific and experimental medicine. The ethical and legal concept of informed consent of the patient did not develop out of medicine but was rather a social reaction to the negative consequences of medicine. Doctors and medical scientists criticized and rejected the concept as a "from outside" imposed alteration of the doctor-patient relationship.

There is no agreement on whether the information- and consent-giving processes in earlier social and historical contexts can be considered earlier forms of informed consent. The majority of American authors used the term *informed consent* in the modern sense of the word only after the development of the Nuremberg Code, because only there was the concept of informed consent defined in terms of a claimed right. Since the 1950s, this legal model has progressively infiltrated the medico-ethical discussion and medical practice. It remains today a valid, basic medico-ethical principle of medical human research as well as of clinic-based patient management. This development was fastest in the United States, led by widespread biomedical research, American case law, and the strongly developed tradition of autonomy that characterizes the pluralistic American society.

Endnotes

1. For example, Dr. Osterhausen of Nuremberg, in his book published in 1798, complained about "medical education of patients, . . . that so many people, in matters of health and life, allow themselves to be blinded by superstition, misunderstandings and prejudice . . . [and] allow themselves to be guided by blind beliefs and await help with the same expectations of a miracle. . . . [T]his cannot be understood on the basis of reasonable principles." Contrary to other fields and subjects, reasonable thinking in the science of health will induce itself at a much slower pace (Osterhausen 1798).

2. The preamble of the prevalent professional regulations for doctors in Germany is the Declaration of Geneva physician's pledge. In Section 2 of the regulations, it is stated that the doctor must respect the patient's right to self-determination. For treatment, the doctor needs the consent of the patient. Giving of consent must be preceded by personal communication of information by the doctor (Bundesärztekammer 1994, pp. 39–44). Section 2 was further supplemented by the "Recommendations for Patient Instructions" of 1990, which take into consideration the Federal German Constitution (Bundesärztekammer 1990, pp. 940–942).

3. Refer to the American controversy in the nineteenth century about truthful communication of the diagnosis. The British doctor Thomas Percival argued, in his influential book on medical ethics published in 1803, that the patient's right to truth is not valid if communication of the prognosis would have a consequential harmful effect on the patient or his or her surroundings. Percival's medical ethics on this issue formed the first code of ethics of the American Medical Association, in 1847. Worthington Hooker, the only American doctor in the nineteenth century who wrote a book about medical ethics, expressed his opposition to that understanding of the beneficence principle. He argued that this paternalistic representation of the patient usually leads to more harm than help (Lederer 1995).

4. The public criticism of human experiments was closely associated with the movement against animal experimentation. In the United States, the linkage to the American Antivivisectionists was clear in the synonymous linguistic use of the term *human vivisection* to

refer to "nontherapeutic experiments," a use that continued until the 1930s (Lederer 1995).

5. In 1874, a 30-year-old mentally affected homemaker with a malignant brain tumor was hospitalized at the Good Samaritan Hospital in Cincinnati, Ohio. After surgical removal of the tumor, a poor prognosis was estimated and Dr. Roberts Bartholow conducted electrophysiological experiments on the patient's open brain. During the introduction of electrodes into the brain substance, the patient complained of pain, cried, and had epileptic seizures, breathing disturbance, and loss of consciousness. When the patient died a few days after the experiments, death was attributed to cancer, despite the massive damage to the patient's brain induced by the experiments. Bartholow's report of the experiments was published in the *American Journal of Medical Science* in 1874.

6. To clarify the issue of cancer transmissibility, the French doctor Victor Cornil examined the breast tissue of two patients with breast cancer who had been operated on by foreign surgeons. After removal of the diseased breast, the surgeons had transplanted malignant tissue onto the healthy breast without their consent. Within 2 months, one of the patients developed an almond-sized tumor in the healthy breast, which was surgically removed for histological examination. The second patient refused to have a second operation and no longer consulted with the surgeon. The subsequent course of her illness is not known.

7. Surgeons carried out mastectomies on terminally ill breast cancer patients and transplanted breast cancer tissue, as in the French case, onto the healthy breast. In view of the poor prognosis of the patients of Hahn and von Bergmann, no further harm can be considered to have been done to them, and the experiment allowed the investigation of an eminently practical and scientific problem, the answer to which could not have been otherwise proven.

8. This document has been misinterpreted and overestimated in the American literature, and its relevance was expanded to include all tuberculous patients. "No American legislature, however, went as far as the Prussian government, which in 1891 enacted a regulation that insured that all tuberculin would 'in no case be used against the patient's will' " (Lederer 1995, p. 13).

9. In this process of revision, the Royal Court abrogated a decision of the Hamburg Local Court. The defendant was the chair of the surgical department of the Union Hospital in Hamburg. After an unsuccessful trial of partial resection of bone tuberculosis, the doctor performed a foot amputation on a minor patient, against the will of the father. The latter, a naturopath, had objected to the surgical intervention, which would cause a permanent handicap. Despite the repeated objection of the patient's father, the foot amputation was carried out on June 23, 1893, expert opinion having been obtained and acted on. The tuberculous infection did not recur after the operation, and the child recovered strength and developed normally.

10. Albert Neisser, a specialist in venereal diseases and the discoverer of the organism that causes gonorrhea, played a central role in this argument. In 1892, in search of a means of preventing syphilis, he injected his clinic patients, mostly prostitutes, with cell-free serum from syphilis patients. When some of his patients thereby contracted syphilis, Neisser concluded that the vaccination was not effective but that it was also harmless. He claimed that the patients were not infected through his experiment but contracted their infection through prostitution. Neisser was later condemned of acting without patient consent and was charged a fine. The state judiciary and parliament concerned themselves with the case, and the government gave its medical and legal expert opinion and instructions, which served as the basis for the ministerial decree of 1900.

11. If this condition were to be currently met in the United States, much of the ongoing research projects would be interrupted. A large percentage of medical research involves patients who cannot afford sufficient medical insurance and are therefore advised to participate in free-of-charge therapy research programs.

12. In the United States, there is a differentiation between institutional review boards, equivalent to the German ethics committees that advise on human research projects, and clinical ethics committees. The latter deal with ethical problems in daily clinical practice and as yet have no equivalent in Germany.

13. The following treatments were used: electroconvulsive therapy, induction of narcosis with ethyl chloral, weeks of isolation and

radiation, whole-body submersion in cold water for days, and induction of suffocation phobia (Riedesser and Verderber 1985).

14. However, in American bioethics, earlier medico-ethical statements are not acknowledged (e.g., the statement about positivistic rights as the basis for the doctor-patient relationship, mentioned in Moll 1902).

15. In the current medico-ethical debates on the Nuremberg case, it is frequently overlooked that the general role played by medicine and the medical profession in Nazi Germany was not discussed. Rather, the judgments related to war crimes and crimes against humanity, as well as memberships in criminal organizations that were primarily against non-German nationals in concentration camps. Crimes of Germans against Germans hardly belonged to the domain of the American war court, nor did the so-called euthanasia crime in Germany (Jäckel 1996).

16. On December 10, 1948, the United Nations General Assembly issued the Universal Declaration of Human Rights, which was similarly processed and based. That is why authors tended to refer to the Nuremberg Code as one of the first documents on universal human rights.

17. The landmark cases of *Salgo v. Stanford* (1957), *Natanson v. Kline* (1960), and *Canterbury v. Spence* (1972) deserve special mention.

18. For example, in 1973, under pressure of patient organizations, the American Hospital Association issued "A Patient's Bill of Rights," which specifies patients' rights during hospital-based treatment.

References

American Hospital Association: A Patient's Bill of Rights. Chicago, IL, American Hospital Association, February 1973

Annas GH: The failure of the local IRB system and what needs to be done to make protocol reviews an effective mechanism to protect the rights and welfare of research subjects. Lecture presented in symposium "Ethics in Neurobiological Research With Human Subjects," Baltimore, MD, January 7–9, 1995

Annas GH, Grodin MA: The Nazi Doctors and the Nuremberg Code: Human Rights in Human Experimentation. New York, Oxford University Press, 1992

Appelbaum PS, Grisso T: The MacArthur Treatment Competence Study, I: mental illness and competence to consent to treatment. Law Hum Behav 19:105–126, 1995

Bartholow R: Experimental investigations into the functions of the human brain. American Journal of Medical Science 67:305–313, 1874

Bundesärztekammer: Empfehlungen zur Patienten Aufklärung. Deutsches Ärzteblatt 87: B940–942, 1990

Bundesärztekammer: Declaration von Helsinki. Deutsches Ärzteblatt 88:B2927–2928, 1991

Bundesärztekammer: Berufsordnung für die deutschen Ärzte. Deutsches Ärzteblatt 91:B39–B44, 1994

Canterbury v. Spence, 464 F.2d 772 (D.C. Cir. 1972)

Elkeles B: Medizinische Menschenversuche gegen Ende des 19 Jahrhunderts under der Fall Neisser: Rechtfertigung und Kritik einer wissenschaftlichen Methode. Medizinhistorisches Journal 20:135–148, 1985

Elkeles B: Die schweigsame Welt von Arzt und Patient: Einwilligung und Aufklärung in der Arzt-Patient-Beziehung des 19 und frühen 20 Jahrhunderts. Medizin in Geschichte und Gesellschaft 8:63– 91, 1989

Faden R, Beauchamp TL: A History and Theory of Informed Consent. New York, Oxford University Press, 1986

Hall F: Psychopharmaka—Ihre Entwicklung und klinische Erprobung. Zur Geschichte der medikamentösen Therapie in der deutschen Psychiatrie von 1844–1952 (dissertation). Free University of Berlin, Berlin, Germany. Hamburg, Germany, Verlag Dr. Kovac, 1996

Held P: Strafrechtliche Beurteilung von Humanexperimenten und Heilversuchen in der Medizinischen Diagnostik. Berlin, Verlag für Wissenschaft und Bildung, 1990

Jäckel E: Das Wertbild der Ärzteschaft: 50 Jahre nach dem Nürnberg Ärzte Prozess. Lecture presented at the 99th anniversary of Doctor's Day, Cologne, Germany, June 4–8, 1996

Katz J: The Silent World of Doctor and Patient. New York, Free Press, 1984

Kaufmann CL: Informed consent and patient decision making: the decades of research. Soc Sci Med 17:1657–1664, 1983

Kehrer F: Zur Frage der Behandlung der Kriegsneurosen. Zeitung Geschichte Neurologie und Psychiatrie 36:18–19, 1917

Kuttig L: Autonomie zwischen ethischem Anspruch und medizinischer Wirklichkeit, in Ethische Norm und empirische Hypothese. Edited by Eckenberger LH, Gähde U. Frankfurt, Suhrkamp, 1993, pp 268–283

Lederer SE: Subjected to Science: Human Experimentation in America Before the Second World War. Baltimore, MD, John Hopkins University Press, 1995, p 13

Levine RJ: Ethics and Regulation of Clinical Research, 2nd Edition. Baltimore, MD, Urban & Schwarzenberg, 1986

Mitscherlich A, Mielke F: Das Diktat der Menschenverachtung. Heidelberg, Schneider, 1947

Mitscherlich A, Mielke F: Wissenschaft ohne Menschlichkeit: Medizinische und eugenische Irrwege unter Diktatur, Bürokratie und Krieg. Heidelberg, Schneider, 1949

Moll A: Ärztliche Ethik: die Pflichten des Arztes in allen Beziehungen seiner Tätigkeit. Stuttgart, Enke, 1902, p 246

Natanson v. Kline, 350 P. 2d 1093, 1104 (Kan. 1960)

National Commission for the Protection of Human Subjects of Biomedical and Behavioral Research: Belmont Report: Ethical Principles and Guidelines for the Protection of Human Subjects of Research. Washington, DC, U.S. Government Printing Office, 1979

Osterhausen JK: Vorrede, in Über medicinische Aufklärung. Zürich, Heinrich Geßner, 1798

Pernick MS: The patient's role in medical decision making: a social history of informed consent in medical therapy, in Making Health Care Decisions: A Report on the Ethical and Legal Implications of Informed Consent in the Patient-Practitioner Relationship, Vol 3. Edited by the President's Commission for the Study of Ethical Problems in Medicine and Biomedical and Behavioral Research. Washington, DC, U.S. Government Printing Office, 1982

Reichsgericht: Von welchen rechtlichen Voraussetzungen hångt die Strafbarkeit oder Straflosigkeit von Körperverletzungen ab, welche zum Zwecke des Heilverfahrens von Arzten bei operativen eingriffen begangen werden? In Entscheidungen des Reichsgerichts in Strafsachen, Vol 25 (1894), pp 375–379. Leipzig, Veit & Camp, 1894

Riedesser P, Verderber A: Aufrüstung der Seelen: Militarpsychiatrie und Militarpsychologie in Deutschland und Amerika. Freiburg, Dreisam, 1985

Salgo v. Stanford, 154 Cal. App. 2d 560, 317 P.2d 170, 181 (Dist. Ct. App. 1957)

Sander A: Arzneimittelrecht, Kommentar, 24th Edition. Stutgart, Kohlhammer, 1993

Sass HM: Reichsrundschreiben 1931: Pre-Nuremberg German regulations concerning new therapy and human experimentation. J Med Philos 8:99–111, 1983

Tashiro E: Die Waage der Venus: Venerologische Versuche am Menschen zwischen Fortschritt und Moral. Husum, Matthiesen, 1991

United States v. Karl Brandt et al. (The Medical Case; Trials of War Criminals before the Nuremberg Military Tribunals under Control Council Law No. 10). Washington, DC, U.S. Government Printing Office, 1949

Universal Declaration of Human Rights. United Nations General Assembly resolution 217 A (III), December 10, 1948

Veatch RM: Abandoning informed consent. Hastings Cent Rep 25:5–12, 1995

Vollmann J: Ethische Probleme in der medizinischen Forschung mit nicht einwilligungsfähigen Patienten, in Deutsche Gesellschaft für Philosophie in Deutschland. Edited by Hubig C, Poser H. Leipzig, Cognitio humana, 1996, pp 1341–1401

Vollmann J, Winau R: History of informed medical consent (letter). Lancet 347:410, 1996

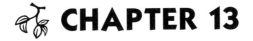 CHAPTER 13

An International Perspective on Mental Health Law Reform

Prof. David N. Weisstub
Prof. Julio Arboleda-Flórez

It is accepted throughout industrialized nations that unprecedented demands are being made on health care systems, throwing into strong debate the priorities and commitments made in times of unbridled fiscal spending. Given the global trend toward downsizing and streamlining of services provided by governments of welfare states for their citizens in the postwar years, these strains on institutions, and more particularly on individuals, have made it necessary for governments to approach the public with two goals in mind: first, to assess the limits of their capacity to deliver services in a manner deemed accountable to structural constraints that are now built into the reorganized budgets of leaner economies; and second, to ensure that the administration of available services is based on public sensitivity to the health needs of dependent members of the community. With respect to the latter, it is a challenge to ensure that procedures are accessible to all and administered in the context of achieving the goal of efficiency (Bland 1998). There is no doubt that some sacrifices have been made, bringing to the fore questions about the role of government as guardian of both individual and collective interests. But whereas in earlier decades such

An earlier version of this chapter was delivered as an address at the Japanese Seijukon Congress, Yokohama, Japan, June 1998.

tensions were resolvable because of the ability of government to fulfill all needs simultaneously, in recent years this has not been the case. The balancing of a series of interests that can often be in conflict among officials, public representatives, professional interests groups, and consumers has become in fact the mandate of health ministries throughout the industrialized nations.

The process of restructuring is the concretization of any governmental undertaking of accountability. However, once this commitment is made in principle, governments inevitably and intractably place themselves in a position of publicly exposing the hard and sometimes tragic choices that become visible and the subject of open and indeed oftentimes acrimonious dispute. Public policy in the sector of health care planning unfortunately cannot—and should not, given the economic realities of reducing deficits and reducing the size of government spending and government bureaucracies that have imposed themselves in the name of public interest—be made in a piecemeal and merely reactive fashion. This means that an encompassing system of evaluation and delivery must be concretized in such a manner that a threshold of health care, reflective of the wide-ranging needs of the community, is maintained and defended. Simultaneously, decisions must be made in such a system that in certain circumstances may entail a cost-benefit analysis affecting minority interests, which seen apart from the general picture could be deemed unfair or discriminatory. The hope is that earlier policies of targeting particular population groups, based on clear public scrutiny and ongoing debate, will ultimately and more swiftly, if the process can be streamlined, protect a small minority of consumers who present the heaviest burden on the health care system.

It should not be forgotten that, especially in the 1960s, momentous changes were undertaken in health care systems that reflected progressive instincts that provided—in Canada, for example—legendary standards of quality in health care, including the use of state-of-the-art technology in all sectors. Since that time, the burgeoning of health care technology and the rapidly escalating costs of training health professionals, coupled with a quantum leap in bureaucratic and advocacy costs for defending and articulating consumer demands, have created a new set of realities in which governments have become almost universally the subject of attack and critique (Williams and Torrens 1993). Therefore, governments must put themselves under surveillance for the systematic reviewing of the costs pertaining to every aspect of the health care system. An assessment of component costs in some cases will lead to a dramatic revision of thinking, with results such as revitalization of some institutions and closure or amalgamation of others. Such massive revisions in the system, part of which include the empowering of communitarian interests, attached to the hand of government, will bring both direct and indirect costs to be rationalized as a right of intervention in the private sphere. Specifically, this means charging governments to question the entitlements of institutions and citizens to use public resources for their own benefit, and to demarcate the limits of unsupervised exploitation of these resources in the name of individual rights. No government in the world remains in a position to avoid these difficult areas of equity. In fact, confronting these questions may be seen as the necessary preamble to radical and effective health care reform.

One of the areas of health care reform in which the battle lines seem to have been drawn between governments and citizens is the closure of hospitals. This has been dictated by the realization that a large portion of the health dollar is consumed by hospitals (Decter 1994), which, by definition, are disease and treatment oriented and which tend to be used by only a very small minority of individuals at any given time. Meanwhile, large sections of the population residing in the community are deprived of more essential population-based health care and do not receive preventive services (U.S. Domestic Policy Council 1993), which could be made available if hospitals did not take such a disproportionate amount of resources. A related argument is that hospitals tend to foster an idea of a health care system geared toward curing illness instead of being poised to maintain and foster health in the population (Clarke 1990). Government arguments, therefore, have been that in an effective care system, there must be community-based care as well as interaction between community and institutional care. Yet as health care moves from hospital to community settings, the administrative structures and responsibilities become scattered along an extensive trajectory of government, health care, and social service agencies that individuals, especially those most vulnerable, lack skills to navigate; as a result, these individuals fall between the cracks. Many of these persons yearn for the comfortable environment of a hospital. Hospitals are permanent and identifiable institutions in any community and they are signposts and identification rally points. Closing a hospital is more than an economic approach; it is an attack on part of a familiar landscape and on the memories of those who were born and of those who died in the place.

Legalism: Social Polarizations

In no area of health have these arguments been played out more forcefully than in mental health care. Along with other reasons given for deinstitutionalization, the economic argument has frequently been advanced to support government agendas to close psychiatric hospitals and to devise a mental health care system that is community based and geared toward helping the patient remain in the community or reintegrate rapidly without exposure to potential institutionalization. Because many patients were sent to psychiatric hospitals on warrants of committal, certificates of incapacity, or committal orders issued by physicians, and because they used to remain in hospitals for long periods, one of the arenas where the battles have been fought has been the issue of involuntary commitment. Therefore, tightening commitment laws has been a way to close psychiatric hospitals. As part of that trend, the American experience with involuntary commitment is enlightening.

This is so because the United States made its mark in this area as the presumed reference point for social change. Other governments assumed the dangerousness criterion for involuntary commitment and in some cases tried to adopt a judicialized or adversarial process to deal with commitment matters. Dangerousness-based criteria could be found in a diversity of nations throughout the 1980s and early 1990s, including Germany, Holland, England, the former Soviet Union, Israel, Taiwan, Australia, and Canada (Appelbaum 1997). Certain differences in the definition of criteria and their application are worthy of comment. For example, in the English mental health acts there was a move in the direction of health and safety, showing a greater tolerance by society for the protection of patients than a commitment to the principle of autonomy that predominated in the American-style approaches. In some jurisdictions, including England, the review structures dealing with commitment and mentally ill patients' rights became more administrative than judicial, and a panel model of decision making was deemed more sensitive and responsive than the contestation of lawyers in adversarial roles.

The American model was nonetheless exported to many jurisdictions and it was thought, 20 years ago, that a triumph had been achieved through bringing to bear a confrontational atmosphere to any case that involved the surrender of civil liberties by mentally ill persons. Commitment laws were passed in jurisdiction after jurisdiction, which unfortunately suggested that seriously ill but nondangerous individuals should never be placed in civil jeopardy, even if they were to fall into grave circumstances of lack of care. In other words, it came to be viewed that the preservation of autonomy should take precedence over any alternative course of action.

The history books, however, do not end with this broad image. Most jurisdictions in the United States and abroad have reoriented their legislation and even their approaches to decision making. The pendulum is swinging toward concentration on the needs more than the rights of gravely ill persons. Does this mean that mental health policy has returned to the state of paternalistic attitudes, which prevailed in the 1950s? Or is there a progressive logic, which has brought us to more recent trends? Before the period of rapid transformation in the 1960s, the conditions portrayed in large state hospitals were substandard, with a very low level of psychiatric care (Rothman 1980). Practices were often dramatic and violative, without any measurable results. Economies allowed for large contributions to these institutions, and disproportionate numbers of poor persons and social minorities were housed in these state institutions.

For scientific, economic, and social reasons, legislatures began to act. This happened also at a time when new drugs and the availability of community services conjoined to make relocation socially viable. After some decades of experience with the American model, the view emerged that mentally ill patients were in fact themselves the victims of the wide-scale reforms. Psychiatric leadership in the United States responded angrily and with frustration to certain decisions by American courts, which tightened commitment criteria very exactingly around the dangerousness standard. The courts were perceived as having put a virtual and effective end to any form of involuntary confinement (Stone 1982). It became a line of social criticism that the jails were being filled with mentally ill persons (Borzecki and Wormith 1985; Hylton 1995; Whitmer 1980) and that families were being destroyed who could not cope with the difficult individuals whom the courts were refusing to put under the care of psychiatric institutions (Arboleda-Flórez 1998; Scull 1977).[1] It was often said during this period that an unholy alliance had been created between the political right and left, ending up in the same unfortunate circumstances of an abandoned mentally ill population, often homeless and moreover violent (Weisstub 1985).

The reality is somewhat mixed. On the one hand, it is true that a portion of what previously would have been a part of the totally involuntarily committed population has resurfaced as a small but significant group within the currently *de*institutionalized population. Arguably, this component has been disproportionately represented by highly disturbed and aggressive male adolescents or young men (Torrey 1995). More important, and on the positive side, rates of readmission to hospitals did not change significantly after the first wave of discharges due to deinstitutionalization (Kiesler and Sibulkin

---

[1]The problem faced by families remains. See, for example, the American Psychiatric Association Fact Sheet "Violence and Mental Illness" (American Psychiatric Association 1996), in which it is stressed that relatives of mentally ill individuals are more at risk of violence from these individuals than are members of the population at large.

1987). Similarly, short hospitalizations do not seem to have been affected. The real problem, therefore, is how to effectively care for and respond to troubled populations, both dangerous and nondangerous, not how to legally define them.

What empirical studies have shown is that even if commitment had been done, technically speaking, illegally, the parties responsible for decision making, whether judges of a court or members of administrative tribunals, tended by virtue of common sense and responsibility to make decisions in a balanced fashion, to address the real care needs of patients in distress while attending to the protection of family members and the preservation of social order (Durham and LaFond 1985; Sales and Shuman 1996; Schopp 1993; Tyler 1992).[2] What has been determined in the past 20 years is a global reality facing those administering to mentally ill persons who are in dire need of treatment while not in any meaningful sense dangerous to others or even themselves.

The first wave of dramatic changes in legislation—in the United States, for example—was defensive; mental health professionals and government planners went on the retreat, trying to achieve a maximal level of legalistic documentation. However, after these early adaptive periods in which there were restrictive and narrowly defined applications of commitment laws, decision makers in the judicial system, along with mental health professionals and families, discovered effective means to make decisions, which comported with commonsense morality (Appelbaum 1997).

Having passed the stage of earlier decades that were highly charged with antipsychiatry rhetoric and expectations of family and community support systems that did not materialize, most industrialized nations are now in a more cautious mood of observation. It is surely not warranted for countries to attack each other through their professional representatives from positions of perceived moral superiority. This cautious mood should allow time for professional representatives from the international community to learn from the mistakes of earlier, eager reformers. They should put to rest mental health imperialism and cooperate for a better solution to the dilemma of care versus rights facing mental health care systems everywhere.

The current plight of mentally ill persons is precarious not because of a lack of quality of restrictive conditions in mental health statutes but because governments are hesitant in giving much-needed support to a demanding and difficult population. This does not mean that the rights of psychiatric pa-

---

[2]In judicial or administrative hearings, however, what is at stake is the opportunity for the parties to be able to participate fully and to be treated with dignity.

tients obtained over decades of struggles should be rescinded. On the contrary, we must integrate the respect for mentally ill persons that has been achieved (often through case law and through legislation) into popular culture and the daily life of both mental health professionals and society at large. Positive public attitudes will become our best defense against transgressions against persons with mental illness.

Human Rights Violations

In the 1960s and 1970s, the cause of psychiatric patients became one of the objects of social activism and legal intervention. Advocacy groups came to the forefront in all the Western nations to represent the interests of patients, their families, and professional groups, demanding the articulation and balancing of interests and rights pertaining to access to services, official representation, and guardianship; the protection of the civil rights of patients, including property rights; and a reassessment of professional standards in giving testimony to the courts or in the preparation of documentation for involuntary incarceration or the denial of a host of related rights.

During the 1970s and 1980s, the world became sensitized to the practices of abusive psychiatry, namely conflicts of interest among psychiatrists and, in the most extreme instances, use of psychiatry as punishment. In the former Soviet Union (Bloch and Reddaway 1977; Bonnie 1990) and Cuba (Brown and Lago 1991), for example, the forensic systems in particular came under the scrutiny of international observers. Because of the popular interest in the spectrum of these violations, psychiatry—more than any other area of medicine—became the target of media attention and public debate.

Search for Core Values in Japan: A Case Study

A decade ago, reforms in Japan with respect to mental health policy drew world attention. This was so because the Japanese government reacted, after extensive consultations, to criticisms that had surfaced in many quarters about the poor quality of treatment for mentally ill persons and the shortcomings of civil liberties protections for this population, which was large relative to similar populations in other industrialized nations. Inspectorates from the International Commission of Jurists (1985) were involved in that experience, and a number of scandals about extreme maltreatment had embarrassed hospital authorities, government officials, and mental health professionals alike (Totsuka 1989).

Admittedly, in the late 1980s, Japan was some 20 years behind the wholesale rushes for the transformation of legislation and mental health institutions in other parts of the world. However, even after the 1988 reforms, which gave rise to psychiatric review boards, very few cases have been brought forward for review (Salzberg 1991). During 1991, in only 0.2% of cases were applications for discharge presented, and of these applications, discharge occurred in only 11 cases (Mandiberg 1996). Given a population of more than 300,000 psychiatric inpatients in that country, this reveals that the social structure of Japan, which gave rise to the enlarged populations in the first place, is well entrenched and has proven stronger than expected. Although this is also the reality of other social cultures, there are real differences in cultural attitudes in Japan that deserve a closer review. The bigger issues, rather than the numbers of patients in or out of the hospital, are the quality of treatment for those in hospitals and what should or could be done for community mental health care.

Some authors in Japan have argued that despite the fact that the 1988 law approved community-based models of assistance for mentally ill persons, to date the government has hesitated to provide meaningful funding (Mandiberg 1993). Perhaps this is related to the traditional belief in Japan that it is the family, rather than the State, that should take on the burden of caring for mentally ill persons. Is it the case, then, that the hospital has replaced the family as the institutional guardian and therefore is looked on by the State as the final and only chapter of relevance? Perhaps it is the case that because of international pressure, certain legislative changes were made but real alterations lying at the heart of the system cannot be traced to satisfaction.

Even if Japanese society could be described as welfarist in state terms, it is not entirely surprising that, given Japan's rapid economic growth and industrialization, the Japanese government has been slow to begin developing a welfare-oriented policy in mental health. As we are aware, there was a steady decline in the 1970s and 1980s in the number of beds for psychiatric patients in most Western countries. In contrast, the numbers have increased over the last 30 years in Japan, where the psychiatric hospital has remained the major environment for the delivery of services. In the past decade, however, the number of beds for psychiatric patients has begun to decrease, and Japanese mental health policy has joined in the trend to support community integration. This shift in policy is reflected in recent legislative reforms associated with the "normalization" of persons with mental illnesses and the facilitation of public funding of community care options, including residential facilities and rehabilitation services.[3] This is now the responsibility at hand and one that is shared with other industrialized countries.

Linking Data to Reform

The challenge today is to define the place of care for persons with mental illness within a tightened economy. We need to determine how we can activate through education, volunteer workers, and incentives to families a proper support system for mentally ill persons while providing assistance from corporate structures such as insurance companies and the State and put together a viable partnership to respond to existing needs (Boland 1991).

On the human rights side, we need to gather our critiques and apply rigorous thought, both in Eastern and Western cultures, to determine whether we can develop and articulate a set of minimal but meaningful standards on which to found an ethic of fairness, treatment, and human rights protections for our mentally ill populations (Gostin 1986; Rosenthal and Rubenstein 1993; Weisstub 1996). We must determine whether there is a core set of values on which we can base legitimate claims to governments and institutions to guarantee the provision of appropriate services for persons with mental illness.

In the current movement toward much-needed practicality, we must set certain standards to wed our ethical and legal values to our needs for adequate mental health services. To this end, we must take a number of steps, beginning with the grouping of those requiring mental health services and identifying in that process those individuals who are not being adequately accommodated. We must assess the reasons for these discrepancies and institute a plan of action to develop both the integration of services and a continuum of care. In our quest to provide services that will make a difference, we need to set our goals and agree to a process of widespread and scientifically defensible collection of data concerning the delivery of services. Through the accumulation and productive use of these data, we should be able to make more responsible decisions regarding mental health care.

---

[3]We refer here to helpful discussions with Dr. Mikiko Hasegawa of the Hasegawa Hospital and Institute in Tokyo and to information from Drs. Jiro Suzuki and Kimio Moriyama, president and vice-president, respectively, of the Japanese Society of Psychiatry and Neurology.

Toward this end, we should undertake epidemiological research to discern which part of the population is most in need and during which period of the life cycle and according to what relevant geographical or localized appraisals these needs arise (Arboleda-Flórez and Weisstub 1997; Olefke 1995). If there are standards that we define by legislation or codes of practice, we also need to accumulate evidence about whether these standards are being met and adequate resources are being provided by government or other institutions to realize these rights-oriented ideals. Finally, we must be ready to reorient mental health law reform to the core needs of patients and their families. Many of the parts of the system are discordant and must be realigned. This approach should also include a well thought out plan of action on those policies concerned with prevention.

With an increasingly aging population and the consequences of shifts from rural to urban environments, we are faced with challenges that need to be directly addressed (Sepúlveda and López-Cervantes 1995). We have come to understand that effective medical treatment must include support structures for daily living in an environment that is more conducive to rehabilitation than a hospital. In practical terms, community alternatives must be coordinated, regulated, and made accountable. Because costs are an issue facing decision makers who are attempting to monitor the application of standards through courses of treatment, there is also the need to assess the cost-effectiveness of the multiple sets of providers operating in different settings (Hollingsworth 1996; Leff et al. 1996).

Transplanting Models in Mental Health Reform

The experience of certain western European nations that have begun creating elaborate community care support services has shown that without unification of extensive government support and community-based interests, improvements, if any, are often short-lived (Palermo 1991). A good case in point is Italy, where there was dramatic movement into the community and away from the large model of the asylum, beginning with the innovative community-oriented reforms of Franco Basaglia in Trieste in northern Italy in the early 1960s (Basaglia 1968) and culminating in the mental health law reforms of 1978 (Reali and Shapland 1986). The intention of this radical undertaking, premised on Public Law 180, was the closure of the psychiatric hospital as an institution.

Tracing the implementation of the Italian law is useful for two reasons: first, because the Italian experience can be related to specific cultural and economic variables; and second, because the politically oriented application of the law was attached to a structure of regional governments. The regional divisions in Italy are both numerous and diverse, and implementation, as could have been expected, has been highly inconsistent (Crepet 1988, 1990). The experience demonstrates that official legislation—that is, the law as it is written—in the arena of mental health is only one marker of success of a given system. In fact, it is in the analysis of the interplay between legislation and its implementation in every quarter of the world that we can analyze the real problems as they present themselves (Burti and Benson 1996; Crepet 1990; Fornari and Ferracuti 1995; Lowell 1986; Tansella and Williams 1987).

The key to effective mental health law reform throughout the industrialized nations has been to isolate the socioeconomic variables that have frustrated or enhanced the provision of effective community services. The Italian "miracle," which occurred in certain sectors of northern Italy (e.g., Verona), has helpful implications for other jurisdictions (Burti and Benson 1996). Sustained commitment to community support along with provision of adequate relief services for mentally ill populations is the same key to the mental health puzzle wherever and however mental health law reform projects are undertaken.

Most important, despite our best intentions, there are financial burdens that remain, in the movement from hospital-based medicine to community services. Infrastructures, personnel, and physical plants remain in place with fixed costs; and with limited budgets, creation and fostering of new professional realities are often frustrated to the point of blockage. Well-meaning shifts from overly centralized structures to the expected greater efficiency of small-scale delivery have not been systematically effective (Hollingsworth 1996; White 1996). We are, in fact, in the early stages of being able to assess the transition from hospital to community, from large scale to small scale. It is in the inevitable interplay between necessary institutions and innovation that we will be able to locate what best suits a particular sociocultural environment. We should always be aware that transplanting models is essentially that, and that unless there is a cultural translation that actually imports meaning into the process, we should remain not only cautious but cynical about prospects.

We may conclude our remarks about Italy by documenting the following: Between 1984 and 1998, the number of long-term psychiatric patients in Italy decreased by approximately 80%. Studies have revealed that in Italy, in contrast to certain other jurisdictions, these patients have not been refound in the criminal justice system and the creation of more private institutions has not been necessary. Small general hospital psychiatric wards and community-based facilities, which involve community mental health centers and residential treatment programs, have worked effectively where there has been a serious attempt to provide the necessary resources. There also have been some strong developments in Italy in worker cooperatives, in which mentally ill persons have attained some degree of productivity. The overall evidence in Italy supports our key point: well-coordinated care can alter entrenched realities in the mental health sector.

As noted earlier, the Italian miracle has not been a miracle at all, and it has its supporters and detractors. To some, the legislation has been truly effective only where people in the culture have responded sympathetically and have not viewed the legislation as a device that threatens to undermine social order or the productive life of mental health professionals. The sociocultural variable includes community and health services in conjunction with families, who remain the mainstay, wherever possible, of social rehabilitation and reintegration. On the other hand, a less rosy picture is presented by other commentators, who say that the insufficient numbers of beds in cities such as Rome have meant that patients are forcibly returned to their families and communities. Furthermore, because hospitalizations average just 3 days, only the most acute symptoms are treated, possibly with the patient under heavy sedation, and the family then must assume responsibility for the care of the mentally ill relative (Palermo 1991). Fornari and Ferracuti (1995) indicated that promised community facilities, such as residential treatment centers, have never come into being and that again it is the family or the criminal justice system that must take up the slack. The social cost of this divestment of responsibility from the State to the family has not been measured.

In retrospect, the Basaglia movement or reform (Basaglia 1968), like many similar movements and reforms in psychiatry (Kiesler and Sibulkin 1987), has been no more than a social experiment based on rhetoric and ideology, not on hard scientific reality, careful socioeconomic measurements, impact analysis, and advance planning. Certainly "the movement" was never based on a sound epidemiological assessment. As described by Invernizzi (1998), Public Law 180 came about when the government feared a referendum for the immediate closure of psychiatric hospitals out of a potentially explosive uprising by psychiatrists, politicians, and patients' families. Yet with all the difficulties in implementation, and as unevenly as the reform has been applied, Italians have reason to be proud of what they have achieved (Invernizzi 1998).

Integrating Costs and Services

Treating mental illness as a medical problem clearly has gained favor, with emphasis recently being placed on the biological and neurological—indeed genetic—foundations of mental illness. The relation of mental illness to physical health is being more effectively documented. Thus, it has been argued that service interdependencies should be put into place and that mental illness should be part of the general hospital reality. According to this approach, what is needed is effective insurance to integrate mental health services into an effective continuum of care. From this perspective, eligibility should not be based solely on the diagnosis of a serious mental illness, because this could arguably compromise the motivation of service providers to treat illnesses in their early stages. A reimbursement structure that is hospital focused and medically related is only one option—and not necessarily the best one. In a social system, such as that in the United States, in which there are insurance-paid care for the wealthy and care provided in public facilities for the poor, a divergence of treatment and protection has been the natural outcome. Indeed, where models are overly medicalized, community nonmedical support structures will be understandably downplayed. Further, an overly medicalized approach is not a resilient treatment approach that is cost-effective (Mangen 1994). The failure of systems that do not include enough nonmedical treatment options supports the proposition that there should be full inclusion of all types of mental illness in health insurance schemes, which, given the competition among a variety of service providers, would maximize cost-effectiveness in the administration of mental health care.

There is opposition to the medical inclusions position. This line of thinking is related to the idea that medical diagnosis remains elastic in psychiatry or that mental illnesses differ both in kind and degree, presenting diverse etiologies and effects. A corollary of this is that we should address the issue of elastic costs and avoid paying horrendous medical bills, lest we bankrupt our health systems. The counterargument to this criticism is that flexibility in an insurance system need not be equated with unrestricted expenditure (Rochefort 1996).

Whether one embraces an overly medicalized or inclusions approach, there is still the question of which group of patients should be given priority. One perspective is that in light of limited and in some cases constrained economic resources, only mentally ill patients who are in the greatest need should be given the same priority that patients with physical disabilities are given. Further, it is argued that patients with more severe mental illness are clearly in greater need of mental health services. This position draws strength both from the practical consideration that there is evidence of successful treatment of severe mental illness and from the social interest in correcting the record of maltreatment and discrimination of persons with severe mental illness (Lam et al. 1993).

Debates about how to prioritize mental health services now permeate discussions about mental health care policy everywhere. Each country has its own specific history and pattern of protection and insurance, and it is extremely important that the historical and cultural origins of the debates as they have unfolded in specific instances not be forgotten. If the unique context and circumstances of a given jurisdiction are not considered, there could be a repetition of what occurred in the 1970s and 1980s, namely transplantation of American-style mental health legislation to foreign jurisdictions, analogous to importation of ready-made economic structures that do not meet the particular country's specific needs.

What is required in the configuration of an effective mental health policy is an articulation of the nuances—in terms of family life and incentives for work, for example—and the connecting of such variables with the orientation of persons and various levels of government to welfare-minded initiatives. We also need to clarify the relationship between private and public sector insurance provisions and become clear about the training and attitudes of mental health professionals, the specified roles and models of legal representation and advocacy, and judicial or administrative decision-making to put into effect decided-on plans or standards. Without careful analysis of all of these factors, reimbursement schemes will meet the same end that misguided legislative enactment did in preceding decades.

Assuming Professional Responsibility for Continuing Care

Our difficulties are further heightened by the fact that our scientific understanding of facilities and their effectiveness "out of hospital" is inadequate. Data are difficult to obtain because services often fall into the ill-defined area that exists between health and social services (Marks 1989). The situation is compounded by the fact that responsibilities for deinstitutionalized patients fall on volunteers, families, and local political authorities. It is therefore difficult to monitor services and gauge the efficacy of interventions.

An issue to be dealt with in all large-scale mental health care systems is the need for continuing care. Long-term patients are not necessarily chronic in the sense of being institutionally dependent throughout the course of their illnesses. Rather, there are significant numbers of patients within any mental health care system who use services from time to time (National Advisory Mental Health Council 1993). There continue to be limitations with respect to legal entitlements and recurrent problems in the administration and coordination of services for these patients. The issue of costs permeates the decision-making process.

We should readily admit that in almost all advanced economies, there are ambiguities about the parameters of private versus public entitlements; and insurance schemes, even when public, have private components, and vice versa. Adding to the difficulties are the problems associated with the movement from highly centralized models to localized units of delivery and application. Within these decentralized units, mental health professionals are often conflicted about their professional roles and are in need of direction and reeducation.

Although there has been a strong tendency to create greater efficiency and greater responsiveness to localized problems, the preservation of geographic equity remains a challenge. We are hard pressed in many instances to guarantee minimum uniform standards, and as the numbers of decentralized players in the system increase, unpredictable and uncontrollable political variables come into play. Critically, decentralization has changed budgetary relations between central, regional, and local health and welfare agencies. Typically, the dispersing of authority to lower levels—particularly when done by a central government—has been exploited as an opportunity to reduce budgetary commitments.

In a recent review of the Thatcher policies in England on the delivery of mental health services, which assigned decision-making responsibilities to smaller units on the basis of cost-efficiency, Hollingsworth (1996) noted that the English experience has paralleled that of other welfare states. Resources have become increasingly slender, and the contest of wills among established and newly created service providers has compromised delivery of care. The success rate of community-based services has been regrettably low. In fact, there is great variability in mental health policy practices of countries of similar economic capacity, even those with parallel universal health schemes. To date, we possess limited knowledge about the effectiveness of the actual practices in place (Hollingsworth 1996).

However, it is still constructive for mental health professionals and social planners to attempt to identify the basic principles for effective law reform. We have already come some distance in redressing earlier imbalances between institutional and community-based support systems. In many jurisdictions, there is a broad range of available services, including not only treatment and rehabilitation but also preventive and educational supports. In many places in the world, we have created mental health care systems that are more responsive to needs that reflect geography, ethnicity, and populations affected by specific illnesses. We have created and implemented programs for delivery of mental health services in less formal contexts, programs often involving volunteers. We have increasingly recognized the importance of seeing patients as consumers of services and, as a complement, families as co-workers with mental health professionals and patients in the process of identifying, delivering, and evaluating needed treatments and services (Hoult 1993).

In the scientific domain, we are beginning to amass data that will help us become more accountable both to patients and decision makers concerning costs and efficiency (Lemco 1994). Agencies and institutions are becoming increasingly self-reflective about how they can most effectively interact with other units in the mental health care system. Of course, resolving many of these problems is made easier when there is a single-payer system. Despite the aforementioned tensions engendered by the reduction of health budgets, there is also a positive dimension in some programs of social and legal reform: an emerging willingness of professional parties in the system to agree that given financial constraints, there is no choice but to act according to principles of openness and cooperation, to develop wide-ranging solutions rather than attend to the short-term needs of specific groups.

We must identify the best institutions and practices that realize specific aims and objectives within mental health care systems. The process is likely to yield key elements that are necessary, although insufficient in and of themselves, to constitute an effective and morally responsible mental health apparatus. There is widespread agreement that the best case management programs are those that are assertive and community based (Holloway and Carson 1998). For persons needing continuing care, crisis programs must be implemented in the least intrusive manner. In the area of housing, professionally supervised community residences must be provided with the assurance of necessary government support. To implement these policies, governments must fashion statutory guidelines that ensure access to mental health services.

Treatment alternatives must be continually clarified and evaluated. We should avoid either-or thinking and rhetorical or ideologically driven critiques in periods of frustration. We have come to learn that it is through a balance of hospital and community services that patients will receive proper attention. We must now develop the appropriate structure to accommodate the diverse needs of specific regions and populations. We should be wary of any moves toward decentralization that contribute to the erosion of central and authoritative standards that carry ethical significance. Effectiveness at the expense of professional standards should be questioned and confronted. Welfare-oriented nations such as Canada still carry the responsibility of maintaining standards that can be applied consistently for the benefit of all citizens. If there are exceptions, they should be made only on an experimental or short-term basis, because mental health care and services form part of a country's moral responsibility. However, we must avoid the pitfalls of excessive concentration of power at the center, which may be overly bureaucratic and too rigid to respond to consumer needs.

It must be the objective of mental health law reform in the twenty-first century to involve consumers of mental health services to the greatest extent possible, as makers of decisions, to the best of their abilities, affecting their own well-being and their eventual reentry into society as productive citizens (Fisher 1994). Programs of funding for leadership training that will assist consumers in articulating their concerns must be implemented. Mental health professionals, as well as the public, must be educated about the activities of consumers in a nonstigmatizing manner. Families must be encouraged to be engaged in all of the processes affecting their mentally ill family members. Programs that support the employment of mentally ill persons must be developed and continually be evaluated for their pertinence in psychosocial rehabilitation.

In mental health law reform, there should be no one model for creating a mental health authority. Each social-political-economic culture must find its route to implement a plan for distributing responsibility between central and decentralized bodies. Much will depend on the character and type of decision makers who are placed at various levels in any given system of decision making and delivery. Integrating systems both vertically and horizontally remains a challenge for planners everywhere. First and foremost, we must be able to reflect internally on our own systems, both in the light of universally shared values and on the basis of relevant criteria that emerge from established practices and norms of a particular environment (González Uzcátegui and Levav 1991). Mental health professionals should have a sense of moral obligation in searching for the standards and goals that will motivate their responses to suggested changes from government. Government, on the other hand, must strive to preserve professional standards in the mental health care system. Cost cutting should be challenged by responsible agents of the mental health care system in all professional quarters. Mental health professionals must form alliances with their legal counterparts, consumers, and appropriate political forces, including the media, to demand of government and other corporate interests, such as insurance enterprises, that high-quality services be protected.

Such partnerships can, over time, build toward an international consensus of values that will enhance the prospects within both the public and private sectors of improving the quality of life for persons in need of mental health services. We must give our best efforts to devising the ways to ensure continuity of care that is responsive and sensitive to specific patients in specific contexts and tied to real reference points in mental health services. Continuity without integration would be tantamount to defeat in achieving our collective objectives. We have arrived at a stage in mental health policy where reasonable persons should not come to unreasonable disagreements about what the key issues are that need to be addressed. Hospital care remains a necessity, but hospitals without community services will regress to asylums. Community services without public support will fall by the wayside.

The dialogue between government and mental health professionals carries the moral burden of redressing the wrongs that have been done to mentally ill persons over centuries. In fact, it will be the measure of our civility that we devote ourselves to finding basic principles for creating legislation that will allow professionals to use their training and best resources to integrate not only mental health services but also persons with mental illness into society.

References

American Psychiatric Association: Violence and Mental Illness (APA Fact Sheet Series). Washington, DC, American Psychiatric Association, 1996 (Available at http://www.appi.org.)

Appelbaum P: Almost a revolution: an international perspective on the law of involuntary commitment. J Am Acad Psychiatry Law 25:135–147, 1997

Arboleda-Flórez J: Mental illness and violence: an epidemiological appraisal of the evidence. Can J Psychiatry 43:989–996, 1998

Arboleda-Flórez J, Weisstub DN: Epidemiological research with vulnerable populations. Acta Psychiatrica Belgica 97:125–165, 1997

Basaglia F: L'Instituzione negata. Turin, Italy, Einaudi, 1968

Bland RC: Psychiatry and the burden of mental illness. Can J Psychiatry 43:801–810, 1998

Bloch S, Reddaway P: Psychiatric Terror: How Soviet Psychiatry Is Used to Suppress Dissent. New York, Basic Books, 1977

Boland P: Making Managed Healthcare Work. New York, McGraw-Hill, 1991

Bonnie RJ: Soviet psychiatry and human rights: reflections on the report of the U.S. delegation. Law, Medicine and Health Care 18:123–131, 1990

Borzecki M, Wormith JS: The criminalization of psychiatrically ill people: a review with a Canadian perspective. Psychiatric Journal of the University of Ottawa 10:241–247, 1985

Brown CJ, Lago AM: The Politics of Psychiatry in Revolutionary Cuba. New Brunswick, Transaction Publishers, 1991

Burti L, Benson PR: Psychiatric reform in Italy: developments since 1978. Int J Law Psychiatry 19:373–390, 1996

Clarke JN: Health, Illness, and Medicine in Canada. Toronto, McClelland & Stewart, 1990

Crepet P: The Italian mental health reform nine years on. Acta Psychiatr Scand 77:515–523, 1988

Crepet P: A transition period in psychiatric care in Italy: ten years after the reform. Br J Psychiatry 156:27–36, 1990

Decter MB: Healing Medicare. Toronto, McGilligan Books, 1994

Durham M, LaFond JQ: The empirical consequences and policy implications of broadening the statutory criteria for civil commitment. Yale Law and Policy Review 3:395–446, 1985

Fisher DB: Health care reform based on an empowerment model of recovery by people with psychiatric disabilities. Hospital and Community Psychiatry 45:913–915, 1994

Fornari U, Ferracuti S: Special judicial psychiatric hospitals in Italy and the shortcomings of the mental health law. The Journal of Forensic Psychiatry 6:381–392, 1995

González Uzcátegui R, Levav I: Reestructuración de la atención psiquiátrica: bases conceptuales y guías para su implementación. Washington, DC, Organización Panamericana de la Salud, 1991

Gostin L: Human rights in mental health: a proposal for five international standards based upon the Japanese experience. Int J Law Psychiatry 10:353–368, 1986

Hollingsworth EJ: Mental health services in England: the 1990s. Int J Law Psychiatry 19:309–326, 1996

Holloway F, Carson J: Intensive care management for the severely mentally ill. Br J Psychiatry 192:19–22, 1998

Hoult J: Comprehensive services for the mentally ill. Current Opinion in Psychiatry 6:238–245, 1993

Hylton J: Care or Control: Health or Criminal Justice Options for the Long-Term Seriously Mentally Ill (Social Action Series). Toronto, CMHA National Office, 1995, pp 1–12

Harding TW, Schneider J, Vizotsky HM: Human Rights and Mental Patients in Japan. Geneva, Switzerland, International Commission of Jurists, 1985

Invernizzi G: Community psychiatry in Italy. New Trends in Experimental and Clinical Psychiatry 14:89–92, 1998

Kiesler CA, Sibulkin AE: Mental Hospitalization—Myths and Facts About a National Crisis. Newbury Park, CA, Sage, 1987

Lam HR, Goldfinger SM, Greenfeld D, et al: Ensuring services for persons with chronic mental illness under national health care reform. Hospital and Community Psychiatry 44:545–546, 1993

Leff J, Trieman N, Gooch C: Team for the Assessment of Psychiatric Service (TAPS) Project 33: prospective follow-up study of long-stay patients discharged from two psychiatric hospitals. Am J Psychiatry 153:1318–1324, 1996

Lemco J (ed): National Health Care. Ann Arbor, University of Michigan Press, 1994

Lowell AM: The paradoxes of reform: re-evaluating Italy's mental health law of 1978. Hospital and Community Psychiatry 37:802–808, 1986

Mandiberg J: Between a rock and a hard place: the mental health system in Japan, in Innovations in Japanese Mental Health Services. Edited by Mandiberg J. San Francisco, CA, Jossey-Bass, 1993, pp 3–12

Mandiberg J: The Japanese mental health system and law: social and structural impediments to reform. Int J Law Psychiatry 19:413–436, 1996

Mangen SP: "Continuing care": an emerging issue in European mental health policy. Int J Soc Psychiatry 40:235–245, 1994

Marks I: The gap between research and policy in mental health care. J R Soc Med 82:514–517, 1989

National Advisory Mental Health Council: Health care reform for Americans with severe mental illness. Am J Psychiatry 150:1447–1465, 1993

Olefke DM (ed): Epidemiology and the Delivery of Health Care Services. New York, Plenum, 1995

Palermo GB: The 1978 Italian mental health law—a personal evaluation: a review. J R Soc Med 84:99–102, 1991

Reali M, Shapland J: Breaking down barriers: the work of the Community Mental Health Service of Trieste in the prison and judicial settings. Int J Law Psychiatry 8:395–412, 1986

Rochefort D: Mental health reform and inclusion of the mentally ill: dilemmas of U.S. policy-making. Int J Law Psychiatry 19:223–238, 1996

Rosenthal E, Rubenstein LS: International human rights advocacy under the "Principles for the Protection of Persons With Mental Illness." Int J Law Psychiatry 16:257–300, 1993

Rothman DJ: Conscience and Convenience: The Asylum and Its Alternatives in Progressive America. Boston, MA, Little, Brown, 1980

Sales BD, Shuman DW: The newly emerging mental health law, in Law, Mental Health, and Mental Disorder. Edited by Sales BD, Shuman DW. Pacific Grove, CA, Brooks/Cole Publishing, 1996, pp 2–14

Salzberg SM: Japan's new mental health law: more light shed on dark places? Int J Law Psychiatry 14:137–168, 1991

Schopp RF: Therapeutic jurisprudence and conflicts among values in mental health law. Behav Sci Law 11:31–45, 1993

Scull A: Decarceration, Community Treatment and the Deviant: A Radical View. Englewood Cliffs, NJ, Prentice-Hall, 1977

Sepúlveda J, López-Cervantes M: Health conditions in North America, in Health Systems in an Era of Globalization. Edited by Freeman P, Gómez-Dantés O, Frenk J. Washington, DC, U.S. National Academy of Sciences and Mexico City, Mexico, National Academy of Medicine, 1995, pp 80–83

Stone A: Psychiatric abuse and legal reform: two ways to make a bad situation worse. Int J Law Psychiatry 5:9–28, 1982

Tansella M, Williams P: The Italian experience and its implications. Psychol Med 17:283–289, 1987

Torrey EF: Surviving Schizophrenia. New York, HarperCollins, 1995

Totsuka E: The changing face of mental health legislation in Japan. International Commission of Jurists Review 42:67–81, 1989

Tyler TR: The psychological consequences of judicial procedures: implications for civil commitment hearings. Southern Methodist University Law Review 46:433–445, 1992

U.S. Domestic Policy Council: The President's Health Security Plan: The Complete Draft and Final Reports of the White House Domestic Policy Council. New York, Times Books, 1993

Weisstub DN: Le droit et la psychiatrie dans leur problématique commune. McGill Law Journal 30:221–265, 1985

Weisstub DN: The cultural factor in mental health law reform. International Medical Journal 3:13–16, 1996

White D: A balancing act: mental health policy-making in Quebec. Int J Law Psychiatry 19:289–308, 1996

Whitmer GE: From hospitals to jails: the fate of California's deinstitutionalized mentally ill. Am J Orthopsychiatry 50:65–75, 1980

Williams FJ, Torrens PR (eds): Introduction to Health Services, 4th Edition. Albany, NY, Delmar, 1993

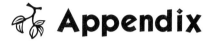 Appendix

The Declaration of Madrid

The declaration was approved by the General Assembly of the WORLD PSYCHIATRIC ASSOCIATION in Madrid, Spain, on August 25, 1996.

In 1977, the World Psychiatric Association approved the Declaration of Hawaii, setting out ethical guidelines for the practice of psychiatry. The Declaration was updated in Vienna in 1983. To reflect the impact of changing social attitudes and new medical developments on the psychiatric profession, the World Psychiatric Association has once again examined and revised some of these ethical standards.

Medicine is both a healing art and a science. The dynamics of this combination are best reflected in psychiatry, the branch of medicine that specializes in the care and protection of those who are ill and infirm because of a mental disorder or impairment. Although there may be cultural, social, and national differences, the need for ethical conduct and continual review of ethical standards is universal.

As practitioners of medicine, psychiatrists must be aware of the ethical implications of being a physician and of the specific ethical demands of the specialty of psychiatry. As members of society, psychiatrists must advocate for fair and equal treatment of the mentally ill, for social justice and equity for all.

Ethical behavior is based on psychiatrists' individual sense of responsibility towards the patient and their judgement in determining what is correct and appropriate conduct. External standards and influences such as professional codes of conduct, the study of ethics, or the rule of law by themselves will not guarantee the ethical practice of medicine.

Psychiatrists should, at all times, keep in mind the boundaries of the psychiatrist-patient relationship, and be guided primarily by the respect for patients and concern for their welfare and integrity.

It is in this spirit that the World Psychiatric Association approved by the General Assembly, on August 25, 1996, the following ethical standards that should govern the conduct of psychiatrists worldwide.

1. Psychiatry is a medical discipline concerned with the provision of the best treatment for mental disorders; with the rehabilitation of individuals suffering from mental illness; and with the promotion of mental health. Psychiatrists serve patients by providing the best therapy available consistent with accepted scientific knowledge and ethical principles. Psychiatrists should devise therapeutic interventions that are least restrictive to the freedom of the patient and seek advice in areas of their work about which they do not have primary expertise. While doing so, psychiatrists should be aware of and concerned with the equitable allocation of health resources.

2. It is the duty of psychiatrists to keep abreast of scientific developments of the specialty and to convey updated knowledge to others. Psychiatrists trained in research should seek to advance the scientific frontiers of psychiatry.

3. The patient should be accepted as a partner by right in [the] therapeutic process. The therapist-patient relationship must be based on mutual trust and respect to allow the patient to make free and informed decisions. It is the duty of psychiatrists to provide the patient with relevant information so as to empower the patient to come to a rational decision according to his or her personal values and preferences.

4. When the patient is incapacitated and/or unable to exercise proper judgement because of a mental disorder, the psychiatrists should consult with the family and, if appropriate, seek legal counsel, to safeguard the human dignity and the legal right of the patient. No treatment should be provided against the patient's will, unless withholding treatment would endanger the life of the patient and/or those who surround him or her. Treatment must always be in the best interest of the patient.

5. When psychiatrists are requested to assess a person, it is their duty first to inform and advise the person being assessed about the purpose of the intervention, the use of the findings, and the possible repercussions of the assessment. This is particularly important when the psychiatrists are involved in third party situations.

6. Information obtained in the therapeutic relationship should be kept in confidence and used, only and exclusively, for the purpose of improving the mental health of the patient. Psychiatrists are prohibited from making use of such information for personal reasons, or financial or academic benefits. Breach of confidentiality may only be appropriate when serious physical or mental harm to the patient or to the third person could ensue if confidentiality were maintained; in these circumstances, psychiatrists should, whenever possible, first advise the patient about the action to be taken.

7. Research that is not conducted in accordance with the canons of science is unethical. Research activities should be approved by an appropriately constituted ethical committee. Psychiatrists should follow national and international rules for the conduct of research. Only individuals properly trained for research should undertake or direct it. Because psychiatric patients are particularly vulnerable research subjects, extra caution should be taken to safeguard their autonomy as well as their mental and physical integrity. Ethical standards should also be applied in the selection of population groups, in all types of research including epidemiological and sociological studies and in collaborative research involving other disciplines or several investigating centers.

GUIDELINES Concerning Specific Situations

The World Psychiatric Association Ethics Committee recognizes the need to develop a number of specific guidelines on a number of specific situations. Five such specific guidelines are stated below. In the future, the committee will address other critical issues such as the ethics of psychotherapy, new therapeutic alliances, relationships with the pharmaceutical industry, sex change, and the ethics of managed care.

1. EUTHANASIA: A physician's duty, first and foremost, is the promotion of health, the reduction of suffering, and the protection of life. The psychiatrist, among whose patients are some who are severely incapacitated and incompetent to reach an informed decision, should be particularly careful of actions that could lead to the death of those who cannot protect themselves because of their disability. The psychiatrist should be aware that the views of a patient may be distorted by mental illness such as depression. In such situations, the psychiatrist's role is to treat the illness.

2. TORTURE: Psychiatrists shall not take part in any process of mental or physical torture, even when authorities attempt to force their involvement in such acts.

3. DEATH PENALTY: Under no circumstances should psychiatrists participate in legally authorized executions nor participate in assessments of competency to be executed.

4. SELECTION OF SEX: Under no circumstances should a psychiatrist participate in decisions to terminate pregnancy for the purpose of sex selection.

5. ORGAN TRANSPLANTATION: The role of the psychiatrist is to clarify the issues surrounding organ donations and to advise on religious, cultural, social and family factors to ensure that informed and proper decisions be made by all concerned. The psychiatrists should not act as a proxy decision maker for patients nor use psychotherapeutic skills to influence the decision of a patient in these matters. Psychiatrists should seek to protect their patients and help them exercise self-determination to the fullest extent possible in situations of organ transplantation.

Index

*Page numbers printed in **boldface** type refer to tables or figures.*